I SAW HIS FACE
BEFORE ME

*Don't cry for me
don't shed a tear
the time I shared with you
will always be*

I SAW HIS FACE BEFORE ME
Living with Sickle Cell Anemia

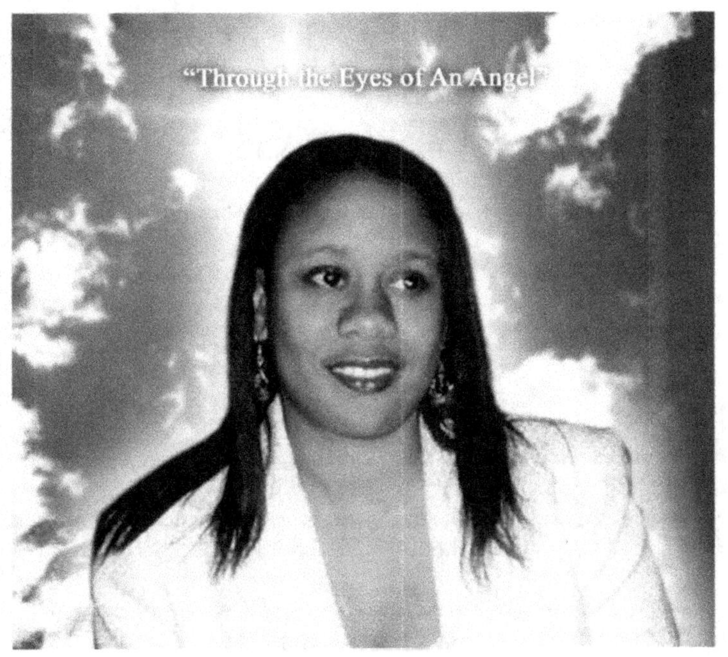

SAMUEL A. BURNS
PATRICIA A. BURNS

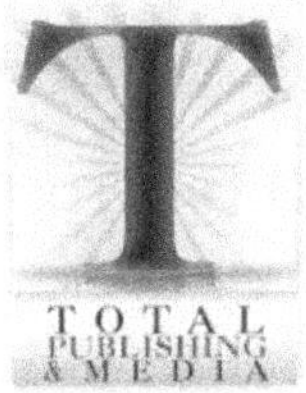

Tulsa Oklahoma
2013

DEDICATION

We dedicate this book in memory of our beloved daughter and sister Heather Anese Burns. A faithful, loving and spirited woman, who aspired to follow God's design - who believed the gift of God's Holy Spirit was guiding her through her darkest hours. Heather understood and accepted God's special plan for her life. Confronting the day to day challenges of living with Sickle Cell Anemia disease was the least of who she was.

This book is written under extraordinary circumstances, for we mourn as we chronicle Heather's life. In writing this book we are forced to relive each astounding moment, each unbelievable accomplishment, each medical miracle we shared. We are forced again and again to evoke the message of our most cherished religion: "God is an all knowing and all present God".

I SAW HIS FACE BEFORE ME is our way of remembering, our way of enlightening, our way of sharing Heather's journey and the never ending challenges of living with a life threatening disease. Through these pages we joyfully join family, loved ones, neighbors, a church family and friends in celebration of her amazing life. We dedicate this book to a spiritual and prayerful woman who spent her life worshipping her heavenly father in spirit and in faith.

You enriched our lives in immeasurable ways.
Each day we love and miss you.

*As weeks become months
and months turn into
years we succumb
to the presence
of Heather's absence.*

*Heather's charm taught
strangers the ways of love
her grace was God's gift
to many.*

*As the love of God enfolds
her spirit and soul
he upholds and sustains us
in this our greatest
time of need.*

God Bless You

TABLE OF CONTENTS

PREFACE

This collection is dedicated in honor of, and with great love to the memory of our daughter and Keenan's sister, Heather Anese Burns. Heather taught us the value and faith of not waiting for more. She taught us to discover what we can do with what we already have, acknowledging even a little goes a long way - and through faith all things are possible.

> *"Faith makes all things possible-*
> *love makes all things easy"*
>
> Dwight L. Moody

This account of Heather's life is rich in dedications, remembrances, memorials and accomplishments. It is an unprecedented look into the world of a spiritual and prayerful woman of God who worshiped her heavenly father in spirit and in truth, while traversing the complications of Sickle Cell Anemia disease. Heather looked life in the face – knew it for what it was, loved it for what it was and when it was time, gracefully tucked it away.

> *For verily I say unto you.*
> *If ye have faith as a grain of mustard seed,*
> *ye shall say unto this mountain,*
> *Remove hence to yonder place;*
> *and it shall remove; and nothing*
> *shall be impossible unto you.*
>
> Matthew 17:20

In this written testimony of inspirational, spiritual, and uplifting thoughts and memories, we share Heather's favorite scriptures, personal testimonial, biography, and the many lessons we learned as parents of Sickle Cell Anemia diseased children. The story of Heather's love for all things good and wise was as integral a part of her every day life as the challenges and side effects of Sickle Cell Anemia; a disease that coupled pain with opportunity - an early death, with an eminent legacy.

On the day of Heather's funeral we asked those in attendance to write a memorial in their own hand. These most precious words of commemoration are scattered throughout this collection. Unedited and not always totally legible, the heartfelt warmth and adulation of so many celebrating Heather's life is more meaningful to us than words can ever say.

We have not gotten over the death of our daughter we are slowly getting through it. Life for us is not better it is different and although we don't have Heather here on earth we carry her heart in our hearts. Most fittingly the Introduction to this collection is penned in the voice of our beloved Heather.

Heaven and Earth shall pass away;
but my words shall not pass away
.Mark 13:31

Samuel A, Burns and Patricia A. Burns
Loving Parents

INTRODUCTION

In the voice of the late Heather Anese Burns

Falling in love with Jesus' message and accepting God as my heavenly father came easy for me. I knew at a very young age he would be number one in my life. I knew I would praise his name and celebrate his greatness during the good times - just as I knew I would turn to him for strength, guidance and support when my journey seemed unbearable – when my disease ridden body would take its toll challenging me and the ones I loved most.

I knew at a very early age that he was the only one who could see me through - from the date of my birth, to the untimely date of my death. Quoting an old spiritual I heard as a child:

God in Me
God in Me
I love him
And he loves Me
I walk with him
He walks with me
We're real good friends
Oh, God and Me

My story is a simple one, yet one quite different from others. My mother Patricia and father Sam met - fell deeply in love and married as couples of that period did. Their passionate love for one another made them the perfect couple-learning they both carried the Sickle Cell

Anemia gene and starting a family despite it made them a very special couple.

Patricia and Sam Burns are two of the bravest people I know. You might call them gutsy, daring, or unthinking – I call them brave! Brave enough to trust the love that brought them together and a God who was guiding their journey.

At birth my parents placed my life in the hands of a caring God. When they learned I had Sickle Cell Anemia they were spiritually prepared – emotionally wrought as any parent would be, but spiritually prepared. God had blessed them with a daughter and if he called her home in twenty years, ten years, or just five short years, they would celebrate every moment of the amazing blessing he had bestowed.

> You have given me the
> greatest possible happiness.
> You have been in every way
> all that any parent could be

Through faith, patience, the wonders of modern medicine, a loving immediate family, church family and community of neighbors and friends, I lived 32 years, 3 months and 27 glorious days. Being alive was Amazing! When rippled with the complications associated with Sickle Cell Anemia my family and I turned to God. Praying to Jesus to see me through the pain - I asked him to lighten the emotional burden my family bared.

As a family we understood God never hurts needlessly and never wastes our pain. We understood every loss was followed by rich gains. Rich gains we celebrated over and over again. My message from beyond is my family's thank you message:

"Thanks for your flowers, cards, hugs,
your whispered prayers and every
deed of kindness shown to us
during this time of our bereavement.
Each kindness shown has been
a source of comfort and strength
during these difficult times.
Thanks for caring and sharing."

To Keenan my little brother, born with the same life threatening disease, there are no words to express the undying love I have for you. You were my partner, my best friend, confidant, playmate, and at times dear brother, my life, my breath. Sharing a life threatening disease with you wasn't easy. I wanted you healthy, I wanted you strong, I wanted you safe. Yet having you in the bed next to me – telling me it was going to be alright – thinking of me when at times you were suffering far more, what can I say other than thank you. For making me laugh, for making me smile, for knowing when I wanted to cry. Thank you for shopping with your big sister, for going on the rides I wanted to ride, for hours of watching wrestling and music videos, for years of memories, for sharing secrets, for always taking my side.

We shared more than most siblings have the honor of sharing – we both learned to accept death as we celebrated life. We both believed in the magic of the moment, despite Sickle Cell and blood transfusions every night. Did you know you were my rock, my unending inspiration? Did you know a magical aura surrounded our special bond? I thanked God every day for you Keenan. I share these lines from Roy Croft to say it best:

> "I love you not only for who you are
> but for who I was when I was with you.
> I love you for the part of me
> that you brought out.
> I love you not only for what
> you have made of yourself,
> but for what you made of me.
> I love you because you
> helped me make of the lumber
> of my life not a tavern but a temple,
> out of the works of my every day
> not a reproach but a song.
> You have done it
> by being yourself"

By being Keenan.

Thanks Dad for being Dad and Mom for being Mom, and brother, my love is everlasting. Like leaves on a vine our lives entwined and I miss you.

Coming into the world on a beautiful September day was magical. With a breezy temperature in the mid 70's, a rush of autumn colors adorning the landscape, and two loving parents awaiting my arrival, my first breathe was the perfect gift.

The spirit of God hath made me, and the breath of the Almighty hath given me life.....Job 33:4

For 32 years I celebrated the beauty surrounding me. From solstice moons to starry skies from misty daybreaks to romantic sunsets I lived it all in spite of Sickle Cell. I was conceived on purpose, lived on purpose and when it came time for me to die I lay my lovelorn body in the hands of my creator and I quietly slipped away.

"I can do all things through Christ which strengthens me".....Philippians 4:13

On January 24, 2009, I died from complications of Sickle Cell Anemia. I was young, I was beautiful and I was thankful for the wondrous life I'd been given. Weep not for me.

For each time you whisper my name or envision my face I am with you. My legacy lies in the memories you hold in your heart. As each new sun rises and seasons come and go remember - that on flowering days in springtime rains, I rest in peace.

Heather

"Only when you drink from the river of silence shall you indeed sing. And when you have reached the mountain top, you shall begin to climb. And when the earth shall claim your limbs, then shall you truly dance."…..Gibran

Biography

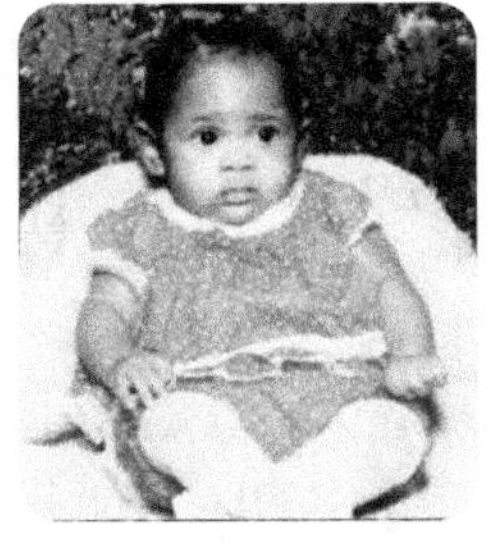

On September 27 in the fall of 1976, Patricia A. Burns gave birth to a seven pound three ounce baby girl. Patricia and Sam named their first born Heather Anese and surrounded by family and friends celebrated this gift God had blessed them with. Not concentrating on what might be and fleetingly ignoring the elephant in the room, they did what every other family does – planned for the future. Knowing they both carried the Sickle Cell gene was put on the back burner. On that beautiful fall day in September all that mattered was the beautiful baby girl they held in their arms.

It wasn't long however before Heather was diagnosed as a carrier of the disease Sickle Cell Anemia. Life for the family was going to change. Surrounded by medical professionals, a wealth of educational and informational materials, a support group of immediate family, church family, friends and caring neighbors, Sam and Patricia laid out a plan for Heather which led to a full, exciting, richly lived life lasting far beyond anyone's expectations.

Heather's early education began at Miss Helen's Private School. Here she developed a love of dance and music - sustained by a talent intuitively her own. Heather attended Carver Middle School and in 1995 graduated from Will Rogers High School. During these years her activities were many. Girl Scouts, piano, tap and ballet lessons and later modern dance.

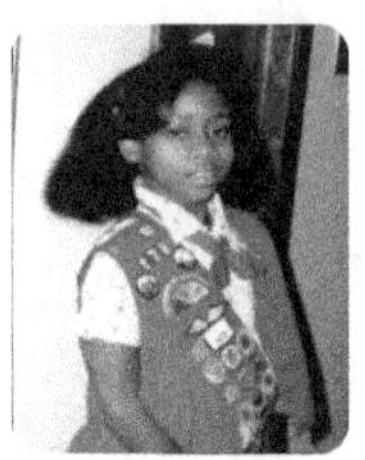 As an active Girl Scout in middle school, Heather completed a Cadettte Journey earning her a Girl Scout Silver Award. Continuing as a Girl Scout in high school she completed an additional journey earning the Girl Scout Gold Award.

Despite the many challenges of Sickle Cell Anemia Heather joined the school choir, participated in plays and dance ensembles, was a member of the Afro-American Club, organized fund raisers, attended not one but two proms and cheered on the 7th grade state championship award winning cheerleader team. Although she lived daily with the disease, Heather did not suffer the full effects until her early 20's.

Following high school graduation Heather attended Northeastern Oklahoma A&M College where in 1997 she earned an associates degree in Journalism and Mass Communication. She later attended Oklahoma University and Langston University. Heather's goal was to do an internship in Christian Media with one of the major Christian networks in Virginia, or with "The 700 Club". She realized at a very early age that the self-enlightening process of education would be a key component in both her professional, personal and religious life.

Heather's high school and college days – though full of challenges were similar to those of any teenage girl. Snubbing the side effects and complications of her disease she was active in the journalism club, in African American organizations, in fund raising, as an activist in supporting environmental protection, and as an advocate for voter rights and registration. She was able to vote and encouraged others to do so in an upcoming presidential election for President Barack Obama. Extra curricular activities included but were not limited to the part of Travis (a major role) in the schools production of "A Raisin In The Sun" and participation in the Alpha Phi Alpha Fraternity's Black and Gold Pageant.

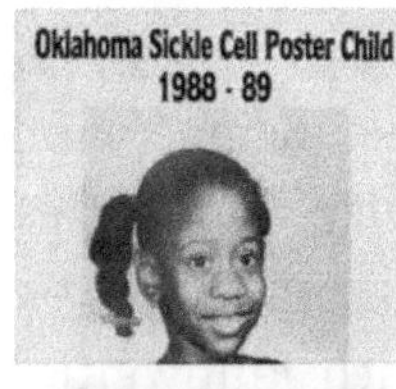

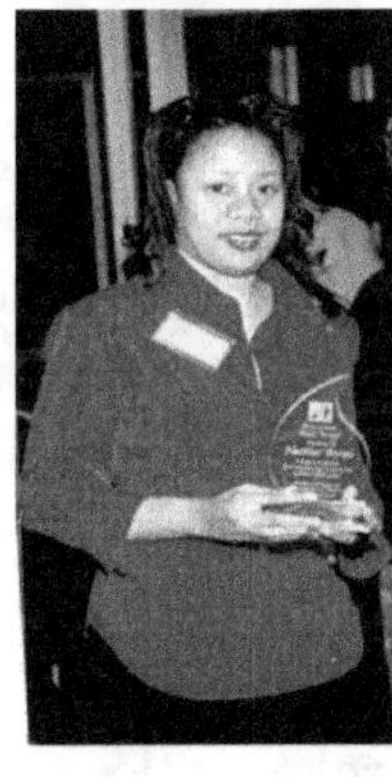

In 1988-89 Heather was named Oklahoma Sickle Cell Poster Child and in 2003. she was awarded the Triumphant Adult Award from the Sickle Cell Disease Association of Oklahoma. Her support included modeling in the Sickle Cell Anemia Foundation Fashion Shows, acting as an emissary for the association through print and media, and being a positive role model to others with Sickle Cell Disease. 1988 was also the year Heather had her gall bladder removed. She was just 12 years old.

Heather confessed Jesus Christ as her Lord and Savior at a very early age. She believed her Christian principles, joyful spirit, love of God, witness, stewardship, commitment, faith and determination helped her achieve her educational and life time goals. Embodying the fruits of the spirit – love, joy, peace, long suffering, gentleness, faith, meekness, and temperance she often turned to Galatians 5:22 & 23, and Matthew

17:21 for strength and guidance. Her favorite scriptures were many including

"I can do all things through Christ which strengthened me".....Philippians 4:13.

Heather was baptized at First Baptist Church of North Tulsa where she was a member through 2001. She later attended Paradise Baptist Church. Heather's love of gospel music, religious musicals, religious concerts, and worship and praise was inspiring. Her church activities included Sunday school, children's choir, plays, tea fashion shows, and later youth choirs, youth fellowship, and youth conferences. As an adult her auxiliaries and organizations included; Sunday School, Singles Ministry, young adult choir, mass choir, Julia B. Jones Mission Circle, youth and children's summer camp and feeding the homeless.

Heather became seriously ill in 1999 during her senior year at Langston University. She had several TIA (Transient Ischemic Attack) small strokes which forced her to withdraw from all of her classes and return home. In 2000 she suffered a severe stroke due to complications of Sickle Cell Anemia disease leaving her fully immobile and unable to speak.

"Not being able to move my legs, thinking I was dead, I felt fatigued... oxygen just was not there"...

The Tulsa World, Aug 6, 2003,
Cory Young, World Staff Writer

Heather spent 2000 to 2005 in physical therapy, speech therapy and rehabilitation. She regained mobility – able to walk on her own, and saw major improvement in her speech. This was also the year she accomplished one of her major milestones. Although her health prevented her from returning to Langston University, in 2005 Heather moved into her own apartment. Teal, turquoise and beige were her favorite colors and she adorned her living space in all three. Having her own apartment as an adult was beyond her wildest dreams. An accomplishment few Sickle Cell Anemia Disease suffers ever experience.

Throughout her short lifetime Heather experienced all the passions and emotions life had to offer. Sickle Cell Anemia didn't hold her back as she moved from childhood to adolescence, from teenage years to womanhood. A love of traveling and family vacations took her to Louisiana, Georgia, Florida, Texas, Kansas and Washington D.C.

On January 24, 2009 at the age of 32 Heather lost her battle with Sickle Cell Anemia. She died of acute chest syndrome - a known complication of the disease. Her life is summed up best by the last lines of her memorial:

> "She was a loving daughter, sister,
> friend, angel and Christian."

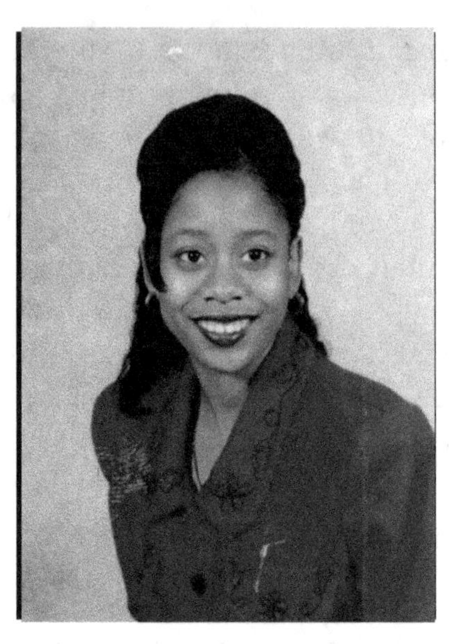

She walked in grace
Led a virtuous life
An angelic being
A child of God
Pure of Spirit
Chaste of Heart
A warming vision
A charming smile
She knew in her heart
She was never alone
That he'd reach out his hand
And take her home
Now she's gone
Her journey's come to an end
Our daughter, our sister
Our loved one, our friend
We Miss You

A MOTHER'S LOVE

Where do I begin my dear Heather? My memories are many. It is hard for a parent to bury a child and even harder for a mother to bury a daughter, yet pressed hard against the realms of my everlasting sorrow there are memories; hundreds, thousands of memories. Absorbing my days and mesmerizing my nights I am engulfed in a mother's never ending love. Cherishing all you were, holding all that you are, in the boughs of my broken heart. Where do I begin?

From the day you were born I knew you were special. Your velvety skin, soft shiny hair, and big beautiful eyes were magical. Generous to a fault you were caring and giving, humbling and kind, respectful and loving. You exhumed in all you did and celebrated the many things you accomplished. You laughed and the world laughed with you – your smiled warmed the coldest of hearts. Your friendliness, personality and positive attitude all added to the beauty of who you were. I truly love you.

Watching you grow from childhood into womanhood is one of my fondest memories. You were my dancer at Miss Helen's Dance School, my cheerleader whose squad won nationals for Carver Middle School, my active talented teen who loved comedy and comedians, my Poster Child, recipient of the Triumph Adult Award for Sickle Cell Anemia, and my little girl fast becoming a woman embracing life and love to its fullest.

My fondest memories are many, yet one of my most precious is your confession of Jesus Christ as your Lord and Savior and later your baptism at First Baptist Church North Tulsa. Your love of gospel religious musicals, worship and praise, and religious concerts was inspiring. I watched proudly as you participated in Sunday School, the Children's and Youth Choirs, Youth Fellowship, church plays and church activities.

From membership in clubs and organizations-competition in the Black and Gold Pageants at Oklahoma University, to your role as the boy Travis in "A Raisin in the Sun" at Langston University you celebrated the life you were given by making the most of each and every day and keeping Jesus alive in your heart.

It's hard to know when to stop writing. When I've said enough or when enough has been said. My cup runneth over with the many blessings God bestowed on me with the miracle of life that was you. I remember the day you earned an Associate Degree in Journalism and Mass Communication, and how your voice rang out in choirs from elementary through high school as a child and later as an adult. I can still hear the sound of your voice as you praised, worshiped and glorified God's name.

Where do I begin my darling, where do I end? When have I said enough? When I see your spirit in the face of your brother Keenan, when I see you in his big round eyes? When I look into the handsome face of your father, my beloved, or when your Aunt Dee Dee smiles? When your spirit warms the tears that flow from my eyes, lightens the burden of my broken heart? Or when those of us you left behind through worship and praise know we will one day see you again.

Your pain was one of my heaviest burdens; your life is one of my greatest rewards. I'll always love you Heather, and carry your heart in mine.

Mom
Patricia A. Burns

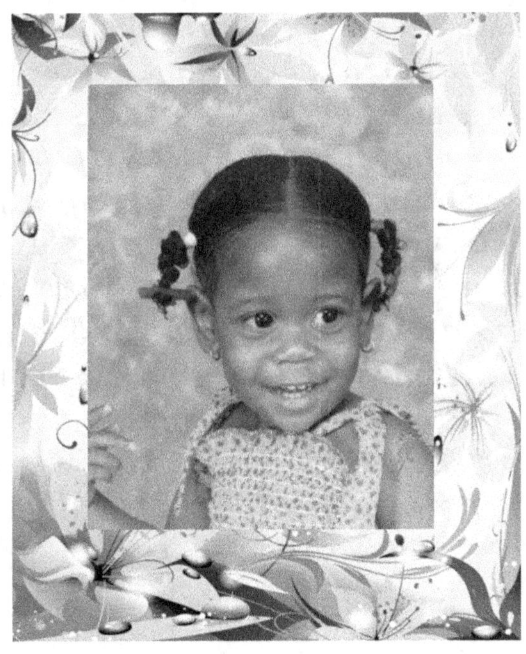

*"Our deepest fear is not that
we are inadequate
our deepest fear is that we are
powerful beyond measure.
It is our light, not our darkness
that most frightens us.
We were born to make manifest the
glory of God that is within us.
It's not just in some of us, it's in everyone.
And as we let our own light shine,
we unconsciously give other people
permission to do the same.
As we're liberated from our own fear,
our presence automatically
liberates others."*

Marianne Williamson

A FATHER REMEMBERS

I remember how her eyes twinkled and her smile widened as she took in the magic of Disneyland. Heather's wings were freed for flying and all I had to do was catch her. We celebrated every moment of that first trip. Every event was made extra special because every moment with Heather would be a memory cherished. I took pictures of her with all of the Disney characters. Images I knew would last far beyond her rich and fulfilling lifetime.

We later returned to Disneyland with the Make-A-Wish-Foundation and she enjoyed it even more. For even as a child nothing could stop my daughter from celebrating life and all it had to offer. My daughter's brevity was inspiring – she was my own personal hero.

Heather loved all the things other children love; family vacations, birthday cake, Barbie Dolls, Cabbage Patch, Christmas, I could go on and on. Yet her greatest and most revered love was for God, for family and for friends. As a self-made leader Heather paved her own path, through instinct knew right from wrong - and throughout her shortened lifetime made me proud. Really proud!

Yet the parent of a child with Sickle Cell Anemia has its challenges. At times watching her take on life was frightening. Following gall bladder surgery with just staples holding her together she competed with her cheerleading team in Regional Finals. I held my breath as she ran across the floor engulfed in the excitement. Ignoring the challenges and discounting the pain. Celebrating and cheering as part of the winning team.

Like so many others, my memories are many. I remember the Christmas I gave her a gold herringbone necklace, and the year she got her first watch. I wish you could have seen her eyes when she discovered the keys to a brand new car that was parked on the patio. We'd put a really big bow on it and had placed the keys on the tree. Holidays with family are special, yet holidays with Heather are some of my most memorable. From infant to young woman Heather was special – no one will ever know how much I loved her.

From a very early age I knew Heather was God's special gift. Never camera shy and always smiling, she celebrated life while facing its many challenges. Getting involved was Heather's way of learning – staying involved her way of living. From Girl Scouts to middle school cheerleading, from modeling for the Sickle Cell Anemia Organization to participation in church and school activities, she cherished every precious moment and at a very early age accepted Jesus Christ as her Lord and Savior.

I watched as Heather's growing love of God and her broadening belief and faith enabled her to confront life's testing. Transcending life's tribulations she developed her own internal clock. One set to her pace – one appropriate for her time. Never confronting - never rushing the sands of her precious lifetime here on earth. Looking back at my daughter's life I recall some special moments – ones that made her especially happy and made me especially proud. I remember her graduation from high school, all dressed up for the prom, the achievement of an Associate Degree from NEO in Miami Oklahoma, her entry into Oklahoma University,

Langston University in Langston Oklahoma, and her transition to life away from home.

Yet what stands out most and what made her glow was her astounding love of all things Godly. From religious television and radio, to a general embracing of religious teachings Heather absorbed God's word and celebrated God's message.

While a student at Langston University, my beautiful daughter had a stroke in her senior year. She failed to obtain her undergraduate degree – yet her faith and beliefs remained strong. The many adversities that tested her were life's stepping stones – opportunities to preserve – to reach unattainable goals and make impossible dreams come true.

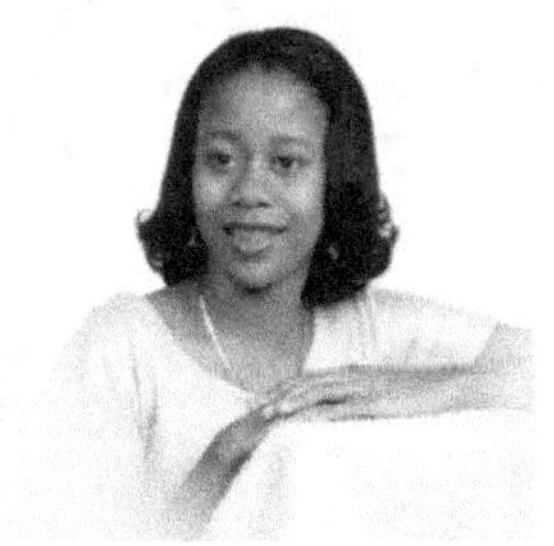

*"I love you Heather
for all the reasons a father loves a daughter...
You're my hero because
you've been so much more."*

SAM A. BURNS
Dad

Your children are not your children.
they are the sons and daughters
of Life's longing for itself.
They come through you
but not from you,
and though they are with you,
yet they belong not to you.

Excerpt from
THE PROPHET
by Gibran

BROTHERLY LOVE

My sister liked wrestling! I was 10 or 11 when I'd join her in the living room glued to the television, watching and matching the wrestler's crazy antics — how I miss her. The camaraderie between a brother and sister is sacred; yet what Heather and I had was so much more. When I lost Heather I lost a sister, I also lost my best friend.

Looking back we shared so much together. Our lives were intertwined like the branches of a tree. I recall a trip to the mall with her play sister Erica and Erica's brother. We all wore our favorite NBA jerseys, hers being the Charlotte Hornets. Heather wasn't really into the Hornets—their team just happened to wear her favorite color. We took a lot of pictures that day. Pictures that bring back memories - memories that make me smile.

The years of living, giving and sharing with my sister were special ones. Years cut short, yet years rich with memories. A family vacation to Atlanta, a trip to Laser Quest where Heather was all in black. My nickname was "Da918King" Heather's nickname was "Heather B-Good"- a nickname that stayed with her.

Heather had a way of making me feel special. When playing the role of a boy named "Travis" in a college play (*A Raisin In The Sun*), she said she developed the character after me. Little things like this made our relationship so special. Little things like this make her absence hard to bear. Yet I have the memories — a lifetime of happy memories.

My sister was the "coldest" dancer in Tulsa Oklahoma!
Before she had her stroke Heather was the life of the
party. She knew all the latest dances and danced with a
group for the Boys Basketball Team. Beyond her love
for dancing, skating at Skate Land and enjoying movies
with family and friends Heather loved photography -
she was good too. I remember my father buying lots of
cameras for her to practice on. Posing and snapping –
capturing special occasions and those not so special
brought pleasure to my sister, joy to my best friend.

The last thing Heather told me was she loved me –
"you know what Heather B-Good Burns?
I love you back!

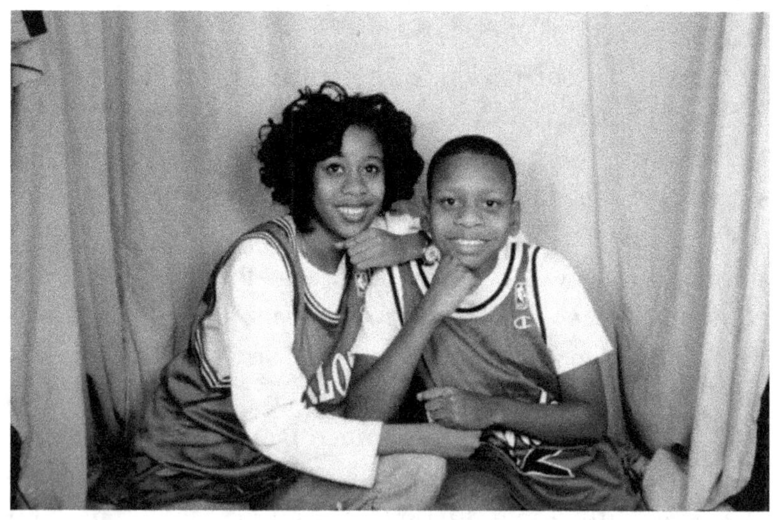

KEENAN A. BURNS
Brother

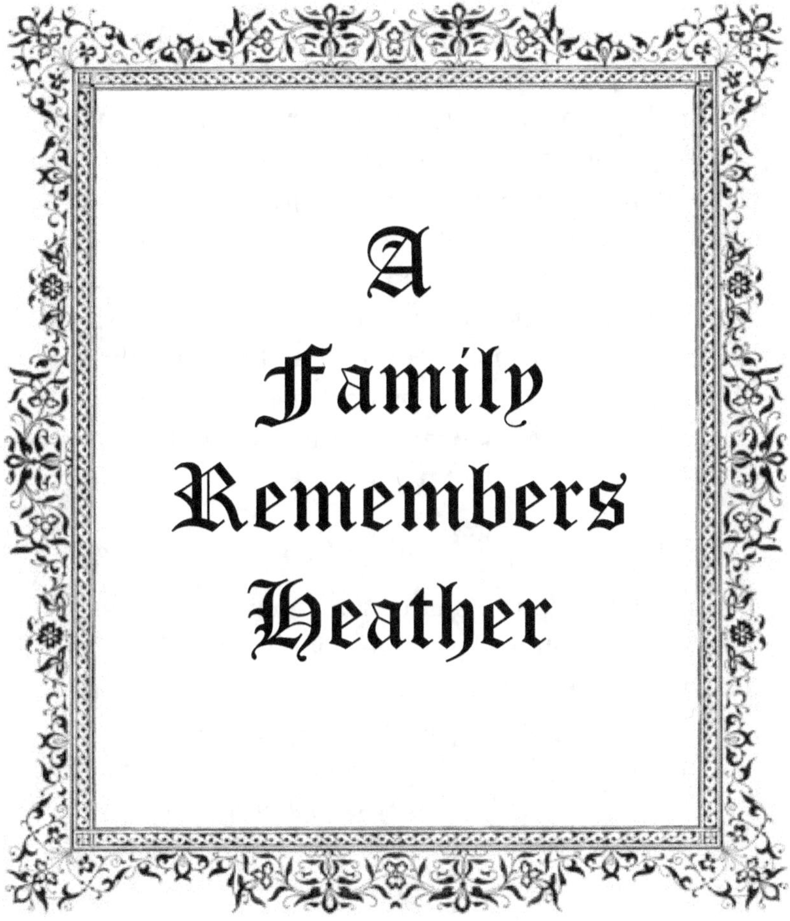

A
Family
Remembers
Heather

I remember Heather as being a beautiful young lady.
She presented herself in a nice and friendly way. Of
course it was about two years ago as I remember we
were on Greenwood Ave for the Martin Luther Kings
Parade. It just so happened we were parked beside her
and her family enjoying the parade and having
conversations with each other. Heather was very
friendly and showed a pleasant disposition. I loved her
beautiful smile. Also, she let me know she and family
had been on a vacation and went to Atlanta Georgia.
She told me that my brother who lives there had showed
them such a nice time. Her dad and my brother are
good friends. She and her brother Keenan call him
Uncle Glenn. We all loved Heather and will miss her.

The most poignant memory that I have is of Heather
at the Hardeman family reunion in July 2007 in
Langston Oklahoma. She was shedding tears as
a tribute was given to her mother Patricia A. Burns.
Cynthia talked about what a devout Christian mother
and woman of God she was. Heather knew at
that moment how blessed she was to have such
wonderful parents

My favorite memory of Heather is when we went to her
house for trick or treat. We had so much fun with her.
We played games with her. When I asked her how old

she was she would playfully say 10 and she was 13. I
love her so much and she love me to.

My favorite memory of Heather, Aunt Pat and Uncle
Sam was when they ran an errand and left Heather,
Tomicka and myself to watch Keenan. Keenan wouldn't
listen to any of us so after a while of not listening
Heather decided we tie Keenan up and put him in his
closet. Ask Keenan, Tomicka or myself.   That is one of
many memories I will never forget. I love you Heather.

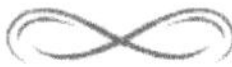

Heather and I were always plotting how we could spend
the night with each other when we were younger. Aunt
Pat was protective of Heather for obvious reasons but
she always let me come over and allowed us to leave the
house and do things together. Aunt Pat knew I would
not let anything happen. Heather wasted no time
getting the neighborhood kids involved. She was good
for telling people what she thought, how she felt , and
she always finished it by flipping her hair. I always
knew as she did that I had her back but when she
flipped that hair it was over. I can't wait to see her with
her hair blowing in the breeze

As a child I never understood what Heather went through nor can I recall a complaint from her. I looked forward to every holiday or special occasion as a child because I wanted to see my cousin. For years we were pen pals, best buds and cousins. Like so many said she always spread so much joy. I have no favorite memory to tell you, but I have many I will remember and love.
You are in my prayers

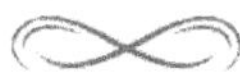

My favorite memory of Heather, my cousin was someone I looked up to as a child. She had so much love in her heart. I remember spending the week in the summer in Tulsa with her. One day we went down the street to go swimming. It was Heather, Donea, Rashonda and myself. There were some cute boys and we were talking to them. Of course like everyone they were drawn to Heather. She was infectious with a "joyful point". Anyway we got back to the house she told everything.
We were so mad.

Great taste in Gospel music, loved spinach dip, a fashionista, loved butter, very petite, loved seafood, loved the lord, Barbie doll collection, slumber parties, biggest crush on Shamar Moore.

One of my favorite memories of Heather is her love for others. There were several times during her young adult life that I talked with her about God and family. She had a very sincere desire that all of her family would love one another and come together as often as possible. She was a spirit filled young lady with a special gift. One of the most precious gifts she had was her positive attitude. It was so easy to love her because she freely gave love.

Heather was one of my closest cousins and I will always remember her. My favorite memory of Heather was when we all went to our reunion in Dallas. All of us cousins danced all night after the talent show. I always thought my cousin Heather was the best dancer. She was a very strong person. Memories of her encouraged me and made me a better young lady. I will always love my cousin and will never forget her.

I always wanted to be beautiful like Heather when I was a little girl. My favorite memory is her smile and her jokes. She always would give words of wisdom when she saw me, "I can do all things through Christ who strengthens me". Heather would tell me and today I live by that. I will forever miss her big hugs.

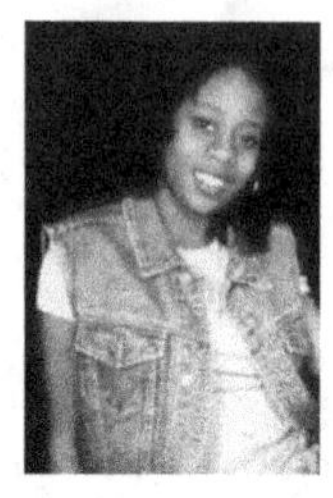 Heather was always a very respectful young lady. She listened to what you had to say and voiced her own opinion but she was always respectful to her elders especially her uncles and aunts and that was taught from good stock. She was inspirational and courageous. Heather fought a good fight in spite of her disability. She never gave up on any task she set her mind on. Can't was not in her vocabulary. Heather lived a short life yet a long one. She accomplished so much. She did what so many of us fail to do each day. She spread the message as the master taught and she did her duty as a Christian ought. Heather left a committed life behind. We miss you niece, hugs, and kisses to you, and everybody else up there we love. I know you all are having a good time. I just can hardly wait.
Love Uncle Oscar and Aunt Shirley

If I were to pick an angel in heaven to come back to earth it would be Heather. When I was dating in the family and then got married into it, the person that treated me the same no matter the situation was Heather. She was nothing but nice, kind and positive at all times. To me she was like a breath of fresh air every time she came my way. Because she was so positive about everything I know God is happy to have his angel back, and she is looking down and smiling on the family. She is happy to be with him to.
Love Always Iris

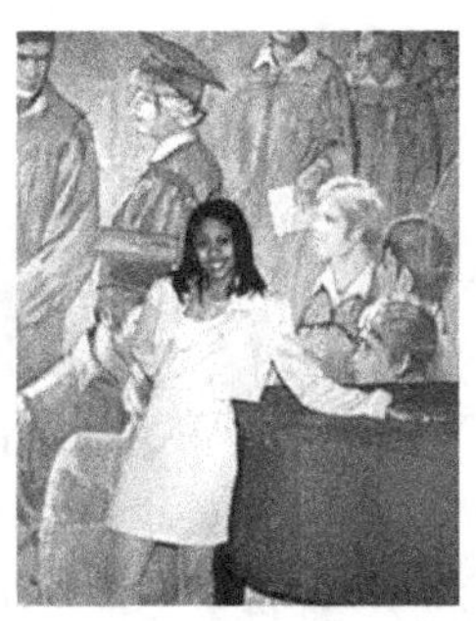

Heather put all of her trust in Jesus Christ. The trust resemblance within the family of God shines from the heart (Eph 4-22-24). Christ was reflected in Heather's life on a daily basis. She reflected Christ's light, Christ's love, and Christ's servant hood. We could all see his compassion, concern and care shining in her life. There was indeed a family resemblance; God's love was truly reflected to those around her. Thank you Lord for giving us hope in the midst of life's adversities. Thank you for being our strength and our shield no matter what, in Christ's name. The strength for our labors let us not become weary in doing good, for at the proper time we will reap a harvest if we do not give up; (Mathew 17 1-8, Galatians 4-9).

Heather never gave up. She seized the moments of a lasting mountain top, experienced quiet time, prayer, devotion, church service, tithing, communion, and spending time with family and friends. When God blesses us on a mountain top "we are strengthened for the next steps on our journey". We must ask the lord of the harvest for reserved courage in our labors. Knowing that he promises I will never leave you, nor forsake you (Joshua, 1-5).

Heather was indeed special to her aunt DeeDee. Thank you lord for the special spiritual and fun times you gave us with Heather. Renew us through them and give us grace to then go out into the needy world to serve others. Thanks be to God.

I want to thank God for sharing his Angel Heather Anese Burns with our family. She was in love with our heavenly father. She loved her family. In Heather's words those are my people. She had two super examples, Samuel and Patricia who gave her a solid Christian foundation and a wonderful family life. Just to name a few; Church vacations, musicals, plays, fashion shows, family reunions, shopping, homecoming, sports events, Black & White Balls and many family outings, which included breakfast lunch or dinner, the list goes on and on.

Heather and I had many long telephone conversations. It would always start with I'm Blessed but blessed are those who trust in the Lord and have made the Lord their hope and confidence, Jeremiah 17 7-8. She did that. I would say "I heard that you were not feeling well " and Heather would reply "Aunt DeeDee I'm not going to claim the pain I told Satan to get behind me and I'm going to keep him behind me." With Heather even when things looked bad, there was always hope. Hope in God, for there indeed is our blessings and our strength

Ella Jordan

To Heather from Aunt Nettie

"Sharing in activities, choir, dance, cheerleading,
modeling (she was so proud to walk down the runway
and oh so good), Girl Scouts (she and cousins being first
black group at the Leadership of Mrs. Johnson, from
Savanna Georgia to march in Dr. King's Candlelight
March to Boston Avenue, a great experience.

I remember Heather's hard work and determination;
completing the work necessary to receive the highest
honor in Girl Scouting. She was multitalented and
loved sharing her talents with others. Loving glowing
Heather, on December 24, 2009, Uncle Felix and Aunt
Nettie will always cherish these special memories. It
was our honor to call Heather our niece.

Heather showed her personal relationship with God.
(Psalms 23). She was a blessed and highly favored
spirit filled woman. Heather was an earthly angel who
made it to her heavenly home. Now she is camped with
other angels she loved. I remember Heather singing in
the Heavenly Choir in 2007, 2008, and 2009.

Heather's growth as a young woman was a blessing
to watch, so confident. At worship at Shiloh Youth
Musical Heather was nestled in Sam's arms and Keenan
in Pats arms. God was there.

Heather's birthday in 2007, 2008, and 2009 is
another memory. Her growth as a woman after God's
heart was clear. Her love for birthday cakes (hers and
everyone else's) is another precious memory. Heather
Anese loved to worship and praise God. She trusted and
put her faith in him.

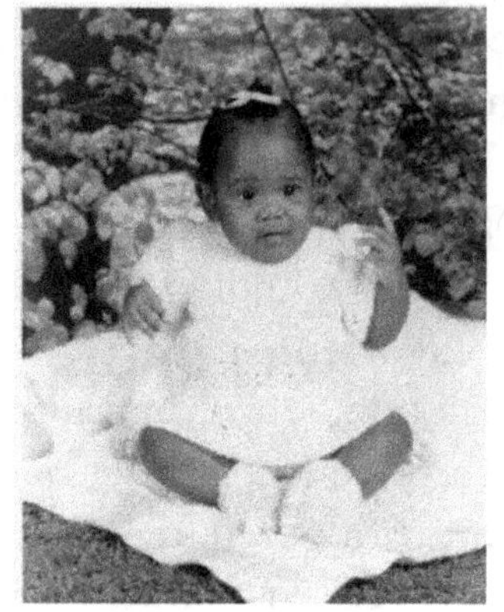

My mind is flooded with
favorite memories of Heather
Anese; her birth so carefully
planned by Sam and Pat, her
name which she loved, caring
for her while waiting to go to
Miss Helens School. It was a
joy to see what a precious
toddler she was happily riding
to pick Trina up. The
excitement she showed at the birth of her two cousins
Tomicka and Tivona, is another memory and Keenan's
birth - her brother - a beautiful moment. She loved
brushing his hair. We will miss her. "

Aunt Nettie

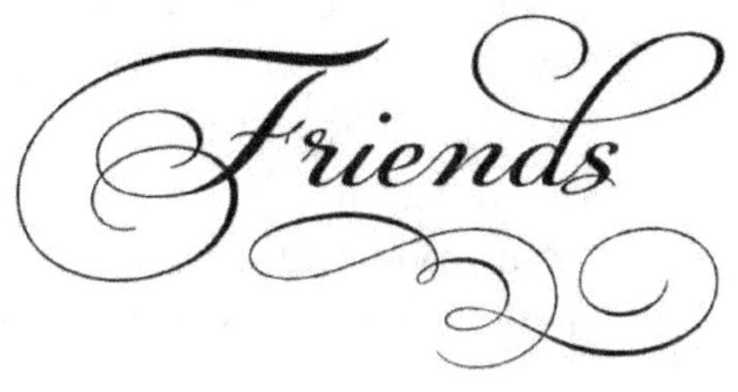

A CIRCLE OF LOVE
Memorials from Loved Ones and Friends

We Remember

A solar dawn begins to break
birds fill the air with song
rays of sunlight drench my path
thoughts of you consume my mind

Your quiet strength
your patient love
the twinkle in your eye
your gentle face
your style and grace
your legacy will never die

Who dares not to remember
a love so freely shared
who dares dismiss your
thoughtfulness
the warmth with which
you cared

As a solstice evening sunlight
begets a darkening sky
I look to the stars warmly knowing
you'll always be
nearby

Sharon Harris

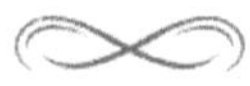

"My God Sister, big sister, friend and my Angel! My
friend Heather was surely a graceful angel! She had the
purest heart of anyone I have ever known. I have many
memories of Heather, but the memory that I hold the
closest to my heart is the way she would handle rude
people who were clearly out of line!

Heather would kind of chuckle it off and say "you
know, you really shouldn't do that"! Her tone and facial
expression was very clear. She wasn't okay with what
was said or done, however she was going to be graceful
about it and keep being her happy self! I loved this SO
much. I think of this even today when I come across
rude people! I try to be just like my Big Sis Heather
…graceful, clear, but not jaded!

I have known Heather since kindergarten, she taught
me many things! I love and miss her dearly. I will
always recall our days at Barnard Elementary when she
adopted me as her little sister - when she tried to teach
me to sing like Aaliyah in her room (LOL), how pretty
and classy she was going to her Senior Prom. There are
so many more memories!!!

Heather, I will always keep you dear to my heart!
You were a GREAT example for me while you were
here! THANK YOU SO MUCH!!!"

Erica Grant Knight

I remember Heather's Love of her Family.
She would say; "to you Momma, kisses are forever
planted on your face", and "hugs momma, forever
hold us close together." She would say "Daddy I'm
alright now. When I was little I loved looking up to
you. I'm smiling now that you are looking up to
me". To Keenan she would say "I'm in your heart
always". Love to her Mother, Father and Keenan.

My favorite memory of Heather is how
soft spoken she was. She truly loved
our lord and savior Jesus Christ.
Heather was dear to my heart
as is Keenan.

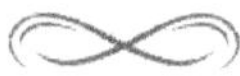

My fondest memory is seeing Heather compete in the
Alpha Miss Black and Gold at Oklahoma University.
Her grace and poise was remarkable. She seemed to be
loved by the Alpha Brothers and she thoroughly enjoyed
competing. Her parents seem so proud and I was proud
just being a long time friend of the family

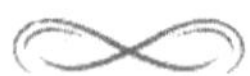

We love Heather as if she was our own. She was as a
daughter to us and we loved her dearly. Sam and Pat
and Keenan, we love you all. Our prayers and blessings
go out to the family. We have homes in Texas and
Oklahoma and you are welcome anytime.

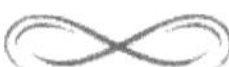

Heather was a beautiful spirit. I'll cherish the memory
of her on the dance floor. She had such boldness in who
she was. She would have the dance floor all by herself
just doing her thing. Now she is doing her thing in
heaven - I'm sure with her spunk she is leading the
angels. I know she is at peace because her work has
been fulfilled on earth. Heather was beautiful with a
sweet spirit, thanks to her loving family.

We had just finished bible study and Heather had
arrived late. She was driving herself so she stayed for a
while to just talk to me and Mr. Jones. We spoke of
many things before discussing exercise. Heather, me
and Mr. Jones did a full exercise workout together.
Such fun! I call it our workout with an angel.

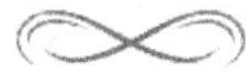

I really got to know Heather as a young adult. She walked in the neighborhood and stopped to talk to me. She was so inspirational. The love of God shined through her as she spoke of many things. I enjoyed her stops. I felt inspired after our talks outside. Our prayers are with you.

Heather always had a smile on her face. She was such a sweet person, always caring and positive to those around her. Whenever she was around you knew you had to make or get things right. She had that aura about herself. Heather never gave up on anything, nor did she ever quit. She is a true inspiration. She will truly be missed.

My favorite memory of Heather is seeing how spirit filled she became in the house of the Lord. She truly enjoyed listening to saints sing praises to God. I would watch her when she visited us during our songfest and when she visited on Sunday mornings. She was a beautiful and lovely lady

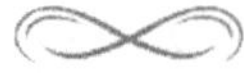

Heather and I went to Carver Middle school together. I can still hear her laughing. I will miss her so much

My fondest memory is dancing with her at fundraisers. I will miss you sweetheart, but will see you soon in heaven

I remember Heather from Barnard Elementary School Girl Scouts and Carver Middle School Cheerleading with all of her friends, including my daughter Jamilah. My favorite memory is when the Carver Cheerleaders went to Nationals in Texas and placed. All of the girls were ecstatic but the glow and pride on Heather's face was immeasurable. She was a beautiful child

Heather and I began going to school together at Carver Middle School. Of course she always had the biggest smile on her face. Through all of her struggles she always made time for a friend and to have a laugh. I mean a big laugh! Everyday she and I would find something to laugh about. We would have a great big laugh to get our day going. How many people can do that? She was my laughing buddy. I will miss her

Heather always made me feel like I was somebody within the church. She would always greet me with a smile. I will miss you in the choir and in church. Your sweet and thoughtful spirit will never leave my heart. I will see you in the Lords Paradise

Heather was my classmate from Carver Middle School Heather always had a beautiful smile that greeted everyone. I will cherish the times she cheered us on at basketball games and also the wildcat wilderness camping trip. I remember everyone at Carver always being so protective of her. She never backed down from anything. She was always so positive. My prayers will be with the family. Heather will always be an angel looking down from above

I remember teaching Heather how to wrap a towel around her head before a shower, at my daughter's slumber party. I will miss her.

I met Heather in 1976 shortly after birth. I was in graduate school doing my practicum. Heather came in due to a Sickle Cell crisis and the hospital did not know what to do. I contacted doctors who assisted them and

began the learning process of how best to deal with
Sickle Cell Anemia Diseased patients.
I've watched her grow into a beautiful young woman
we all can be proud of. She will be missed

I remember when she graduated from High School and
her sweet disposition. I am proud to have been a part of
her life and even prouder that she crossed my path. She
believed in me when I was uncertain how the world
would treat me. I only met Heather once. She was of
course as beautiful and gracious as her mother. I know
she will be missed. The angels will carry her home.

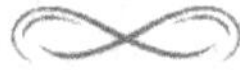

My memory of Heather is at a Vacation Bible School end
of the year program at First Baptist Church North
Tulsa. Heather did an interpretative modern dance for
the audience. I also remember her singing in the mass
choir on Sunday. Heather will be missed.

We met Heather through her grandparents. She was a
very sweet person to know. We will miss her sweet
smile but we know she is with God in her heavenly
home forever. Fare well Sweet One

Heather had a sweet spirit and always had a smile on her face. There were so many times I would run into her and we would stop and talk. She always wanted to know and would listen, to the things you were trying to accomplish. Heather was always encouraging others . I never once saw her upset about anything.
I will miss her.

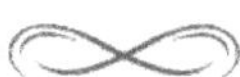

Heather was such a sweet inspiring young lady. I remember when she came to spend the night. We lived on 2 1.2 acres.   Heather was not use to the country but she had such a good time playing. The last time I saw Heather it was at the mall. She asked about a friend and wanted to know what she was doing. She was always encouraging. I'm praying for you and know we will be together

What I loved most about Heather was attending First Baptist Church North Tulsa. If I had a problem or a question she would answer it. Heather would make me see and think about things differently. She and her brother Keenan have a special place in my heart

36

I remember the look on Heather's face and how she wrinkled her nose when I told her I was a September girl also. I remember her excitement about learning to drive. I remember how elated she was about getting her own apartment. I can still hear her say "I'm blessed".
Yours in Christ

The day you were born. How proud your mom and dad were. You were so beautiful. Two months later you got a play mate. I am so thankful you came into our lives. You spent a lot of time with us and became a part of our family. You will be missed

I have so many memories of Heather's soft voice, her sunshine smile, her kind and gentle manner. She was so special and we were all so lucky to know her. I think my favorite memory was the last time I saw her. As always gentle and kind, she was such a lady. She came to ask about helping the Girl Scouts. Heather was always thinking of helping. She was so good, we'll miss her.

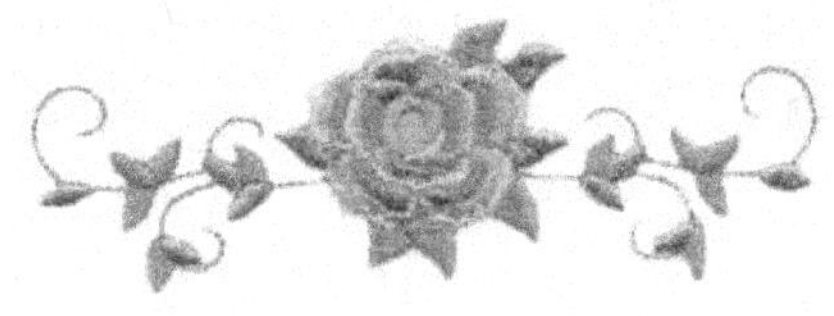

Each time you whisper my name
envision my face
or gaze upon the loving
family and friends
that are my legacy
I am with you

In The Hands of
A Living God

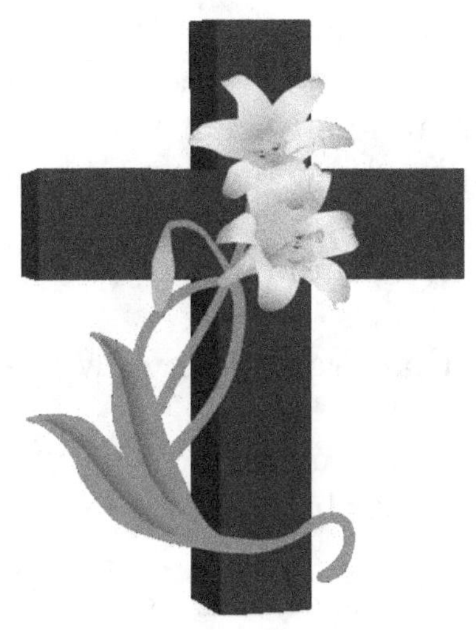

A Church Remembers

It seems you left too soon
There were so many words unspoken
And your absence in our lives
Has left our hearts broken

But through our pain and tears
We trust that God knew best
We wanted you to remain here
But God called you home to rest

You were such an inspiration
A great example of how a Christian should live
Going to college, yet serving God
Giving all that you could give

Now you're in that great cloud of witnesses
Rejoicing in the sky
Cheering us on from up above
Telling us it's better by and by

We look forward to seeing you on that day
When our souls shall meet again
In that great getting up morning
When Sabbath shall have no end

So keep smiling down on us Heather
As you shine in the Heavens above
And we will still press on this journey
Keeping your memory alive with love

Rev.Bertrand Maurice Baily Jr.

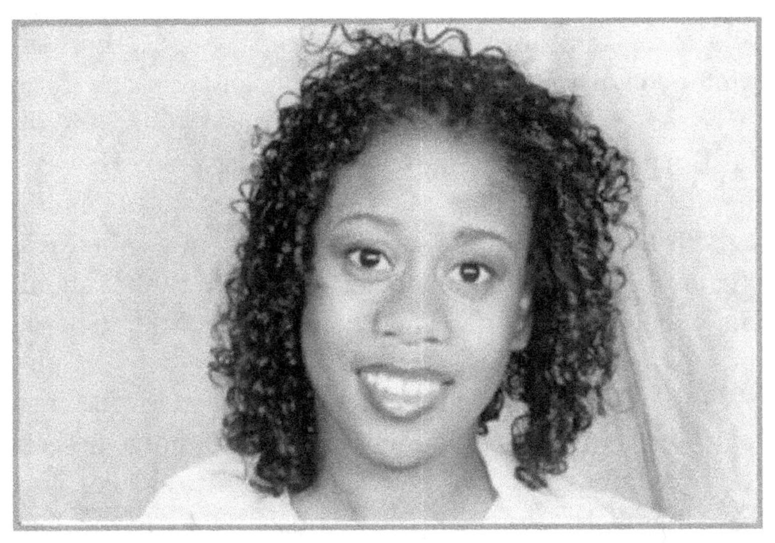

A Rare Jewel Indeed
By Ivy N. Kincy

More precious than any highly appraised diamond Heather was a rare jewel indeed. When she had an occasion to be in the house of the Lord, she shone as brilliant as a gemstone. With skin as radiant as the glowing sun, her smile could light up an entire room. Whether singing in the choir or just listening to other groups sing praises, she was truly grateful and consumed with a spirit of thankfulness. Her spirit was overflowing with love, peace, joy, gentleness, longsuffering, kindness, goodness, faith, and all the fruits of the spirit.

Although she was unable to march with the choir on a regular basis, she was blessed to be able to march and sing with the chorus one last Sunday. Marching for the Lord was her ultimate desire, so this was a culminating milestone for her to go marching in. Generosity combined with service was her strong suits for the Lord.

By the grace of God, Heather was on loan to Sam and Pat Burns for such a succinct second, it seems. However she did leave a plethora of fond memories for her family and friends to reminisce during her sabbatical. Whenever we think about Heather, we should remember that she has gone home to her Maker so she can rest now.

We don't have to worry about her anymore, because God has eradicated all of her pain. So family, friends, and loved ones must hold on to the countless cherished memories. It's imperative we also hold on to God's unchanging hand. Whenever those dark days creep upon us, we must remember our rare jewel that God left in our care year after year. And prayerfully, we'll be able to witness the essence of our rare jewel still shining brightly through our dim memories.

A TRIBUTE TO HEATHER ANESE BURNS

"So many times along life's highway we meet people only for a season; Heather was one of those persons. I remember the first time Jean and I saw her it was at our evening Bible Study. She came with her family. Her spirit emanated with such vibrancy and power, that she simply transcended her obvious physical challenges.

Heather was truly a unique blend of love and compassion - she had such an obvious love for the Lord. The physical adversity she faced, instead of making her bitter yielded a sweetness that was immeasurable. She possessed a sensitivity that was admirable and a determination to overcome which was formidable.

Heather was different from most of us; for although she labored to live she lived to love. Truly she was a vessel that God used to bless others, an example of how to deal with adversity. If anyone is challenged in life by any circumstance; look to Heather, for she indeed set the benchmark standard on how to live life, no matter what the challenge.

Both Jean and I were blessed and inspired to know Heather and we thank God for the time we had with her. We know she is now in perfect peace, resting in the bosom of the Lord, for she has started her eternal journey, one that all of us must take one day. But until that time; anyone who has known Heather can best honor her memory by following her example on how to live life at its fullest, without regard for circumstance or situation. Heather, we love you, and we miss you, and we thank God for the time you graced us with your presence."

Love

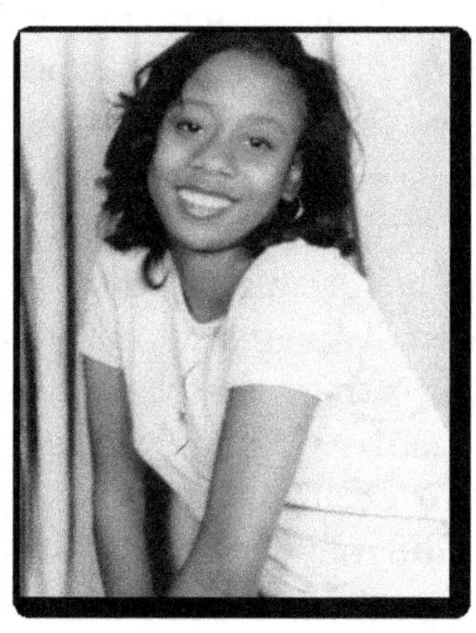

"Blessed be the God and Father
of our Lord Jesus Christ,
the Father of mercies and
God of all comfort,
who comforts us
in all our affliction,
so that we may
be able to comfort those
who are in any affliction,
with the comfort with which
we ourselves are comforted
by God."

2 Corinthians 1: 3-4

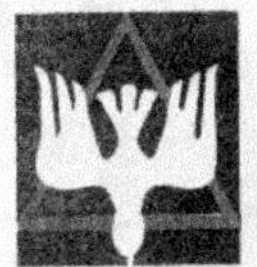

FIRST BAPTIST CHURCH NORTH TULSA
1414 NORTH GREENWOOD AVE. ✝ TULSA, OKLAHOMA 74106

January 31, 2009
Condolence

We, the Ministerial Staff, Officers, and Members of First Baptist Church North Tulsa, Tulsa, Oklahoma, are sadden to hear the news of the home going of one of our beloved young adults, Sister Heather Burns, who was raised up in our church. Heather was baptized by Rev. Leroy K. Jordan in her younger days along with several other youth. She was active with our youth when she felt able to attend. We are so happy to have seen her grow up to be a lovely young lady. We are sorry to have her leave us so early in her life.

God, in his infinite wisdom never makes a mistake, and always knows what he is doing. We thank him for the life time he gave her for she had traveled a long road. She never gave up trying to better herself. God is good and he gave her a good time in her life, our hearts go out to Brother Sam and Sister Patricia for the love and support that she was given to keep her in tune with all other obstacles she had to climb. Her loyalty was demonstrated by her attendance at the services of worship and touching many lives with her cheerful voice and smile. She will surely be missed. We thank her father Brother Sam and mother Sister Patricia for the loving care that she received. May the love of God comfort you and encompass you in the days ahead and we also extend our love to Keenan and ask for God's love to be with him.

Prayerfully Submitted,

First Baptist Church North Tulsa
Rev. Anthony L. Scott, Senior Pastor
Deidre Walker, Church Clerk

St. Andrew Baptist Church

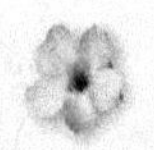

3115 N. Garrison Avenue
Tulsa, Oklahoma 74106
(918) 425-4915 or 425-8380
Reverend Dr. Bertrand M. Bailey, Sr., Pastor /Teacher

Saturday, January 31, 2009

TO: Brother Sam and Sister Patricia Burns and Family

Be it resolved, the St. Andrew Baptist Church Family shares with the wonderful members of this Family in your time of sorrow and the bereavement of your beloved daughter, sister and loved one, Sister Heather Burns. The Pastor, Ministers, Deacons, and the entire St. Andrew Family will continue to lift your family in prayer during these most difficult times.

Whereas the Almighty God has called from this world your precious daughter, we are confident that He is too wise to make a mistake. The hymn writer was right when he penned these words "We'll understand it better, bye and bye".

The Bailey family and the Burns Family share a special relationship, so we deemed it necessary to share expressions of love and comfort to our friends. Our sons in Texas, Rev. Bertrand Jr. and Rev. Choo Choo regret that they could not be with you today, but they have never stopped praying for you since hearing of the passing of your daughter and their friend - Heather.

We admonish this family to lift up your eyes unto the hills from whence cometh your help. Realizing that all your help comes from the Lord. This is a good time to comfort one another, encourage one another and most of all love one another.

May the 'God of all Comfort' give this family strength and peace for the days ahead.

May the words of this hymn give you spiritual solace:

> *"What a Friend We have in Jesus, All our sins and grief He'll bear*
> *What a privilege it is to carry, everything to God in Prayer."*

The Prayers and Sympathies of the St. Andrew Family Are Yours.

Humbly Submitted,

Pastor, Dr. Bertrand Maurice Bailey, Sr.

A copy of this resolution will be given to the family, and a copy will be kept as a permanent record of St. Andrew Baptist Church.

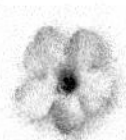

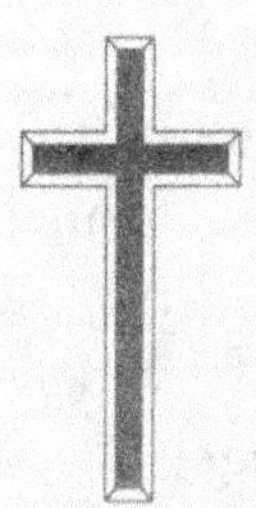

First Baptist Church
P. O. Box 314
Taft, OK
74463

January 31, 2009

RESOLUTION

Do not let your heart be troubled; believe in God, believe also in me. In my Father's house are many dwelling places; if it were not so, I would have told you; for I go to prepare a place for you, if I go and prepare a place for you, I will come again and receive you unto myself. That where I am there you may be also. (John 14 : 1-3)

To the family of Sister Heather Anese Burns:
we the Pastor Rev. John C. Washington and the First Baptist Church Family were saddened to hear of the Home Going of Heather. Heather has always been a real inspiration because of her beautiful smile and determination. She will be missed but never forgotten.

May you always LOOK TO THE HILLS FROM WHICH ALL OF YOUR HELP COMES FROM, AND ALL OF YOUR HELP COMES FROM THE LORD. REJOICE IN THE LORD ALWAYS; AGAIN I SAY REJOICE! LET YOUR GENTLE SPIRIT BE KNOWN UNTO ALL MEN. THE LORD IS NEAR. BE ANXIOUS FOR NOTHING, BUT EVERYTHING BY PRAYER AND SUPPLICATION WITH THANKSGIVING LET YOUR REQUEST BE MADE KNOWN UNTO GOD. AND THE PEACE OF GOD WHICH SURPASSES ALL COMPREHENSION, WILL GUARD YOUR HEARTS AND YOUR MINDS IN CHRIST JESUS.

We commend you into the hands of the Almighty God that He may comfort you and strengthen you in your time of sorrow. Remember that God loves you and that He is always there when you need Him.

We the Pastor, Officers, and Members of the First Baptist Church offer our deepest Sympathy and support to you. Know that we are praying for you and that we are just a phone call away.

Rev. John C. Washington, Pastor

Sister Etoyce Shipp, Church Clerk

HEATHER ANESE BURNS

There are those who have made Jesus Lord by their confession' and then there are those who define Jesus as Lord by their actions. Heather was in the latter; she carried the 'light'; and it shone bright as she lived her life as a vessel for the Lord. She is no longer in our physical presence; but the fragrance of her spirit remains' and the residuals of her legacy will always be with all who had the pleasure and good fortune to know her.

We know that for Heather, Heaven was her final destination' and that she has taken her place in God's Heavenly Choir' adding her voice to the 'Praise' and 'Worship' to the 'Father'. And as we remember this precious spirit, that brought such life and vitality to all who knew her' we know death has not separated us but in essence has brought us closer. For she has now taken her place as a part of that great cloud of witnesses, who are encouraging us, who remain in the race each of us are called to run.

For one day, when we too, cross the threshold of eternity's door' Heather will meet us with that 'twinkle' and 'smile'; and we will fellowship with her for eternity's season

WALDO JONES

A CHURCH FAMILY REMEMBERS

""Heather was always kind. She always had good conduct. In U.B.S. Heather always showed an eagerness to learn. She was all smiles."

* * *

"It's how Heather's face would light up when she worshiped our lord and savior. Her beautiful smile her joy and love of life. Love for her family and friends. I see an independent black woman. I see love for her church and her church family. I remember the excitement when she got her license. The joy in her voice when she spoke of her kind and loving parents; and her loving brother. I will miss seeing you Heather - but I will see you again"

* * *

"My favorite memory of Heather is her smile and the joy you see in her when she speaks to you. Heather will be missed by me."

* * *

"Heather was a sweet young lady. I loved to talk to her. She would come to the church and help me fold programs, run copies or just talk. She helped me out with her prayers and calling during my husband's illness. I will miss her sweet spirit and her smile. "

* * *

"At choir practice at first Baptist North Tulsa Heather showed her leadership skills in getting members to

learn their part. I remember when she visited
Crossover Bible Church to hear Marshall Gordon
Preach. She always had a smile on her face. I love and
will miss Heather. She was a joy. God Bless You.”

* * *

“Heather was a very sweet young Lady. She would
always acknowledge me with “how are you” and give me
a big hug. Whenever I would see Heather I would look
forward to her hugs. She was an adorable person. Most
of all she loved the Lord and it showed. To the family -
stay strong and know that God has her in his arms.”

* * *

“I will always cherish the memories that Heather,
Keenan and I shared but the one I hold near and dear to
my heart is how she loved the lord.
I’m going to miss her much.”

* * *

“Heather was such a sweet person. When she learned
who I was she would come to the church Treasurer’s
Office and great me so nicely. When she learned who my
mother was she would often say how much my mother
and I looked alike. Love and blessings to Pat and the
family, I know God gave you this blessed and precious
time with Heather. I feel privileged to have known her.”

* * *

“I recall Heather’s beautiful sweet spirit. I was really
touched by her attempt to console me after my husbands
passing. She was a loving and caring young woman.”

* * *

"One of my fondest memories of Heather was at youth
meeting when she and Kelly got tickled at something.
Well I threatened both of them. Every time they would
look at each other they would start all over. The funny
thing was I could hardly keep from laughing myself. I
also remember a very up beat respectful child and adult
always smiling ‑ a true pleasure to be around."

* * *

"I remember the sweet but determined nature of a big
sister. I witnessed first hand "you do not mess with her
little brother". Letting the youth choir know was so
Heather. I'll also have fond memories of the modeling
and dancing. I know she had loads of untapped talent.
She was so special ‑ one of God's chosen".

* * *

"My favorite memory of Heather is when we were at Mt.
Zion's the Sunday before the Lord called her home. I
looked back while service was going on and she looked
so pretty ‑ just like she did at her services. She was
truly a busy beautiful angel. She left us so many
precious memories. We are truly blessed she crossed
our paths. Love, and God Bless you."

* * *

"In 2004 when my daughter came down to attend
church with me Heather came up to me to speak. I
introduced them and they started to talk like they had
known each other all of their lives. My grandson was
very comfortable with Heather. Heather loved all

51

people and that smile of hers is beautiful. I know
Heather loved her God.   Claudia

* * *

Heather was my partner in the choir and at revivals.
We sat side by side at the St Andrews Baptist Revival.
Rev Bertrand Bailey Jr. preached a powerful sermon.
We rejoiced in church then and I'm rejoicing
with her now."

* * *

"I remember Heather's participation in many programs
at First Baptist Church North Tulsa and in her youth. I
truly admired her for her performance at OU in the
Black and Gold Pageant. She will truly be missed. God
bless you Pat and Sam."

* * *

"Words cannot express the grief my family has for you
today. Heather; there was something angelic about her.
I saw this in her many years ago and I truly admired
her spirit. She encouraged me on many Sundays. I
never saw her sad. In fact I found myself many times
just looking at her. I thought she was beautiful - when
she limped I hurt. I prayed for her. Thank you for
bringing her into this world. I will never forget her."

* * *

I didn't know Heather very well only got to know of her
just a short time but I can say in that short time I felt
her loving spirit and her kindness. She will always be
remembered. She sat next to me in the choir.

We spoke briefly but what she said is everlasting –
my prayers are forever with you."

* * *

"To God be the Glory. I did not know Heather that long
or that well but I know she was a walking talking living
testimony of God's peace, mercy and loving kindness.
When I first started visiting Paradise Heather was in a
wheelchair, her smile and sweet spirit captivated my
heart. Later she was on a walker, then crutches, then a
cane. Finally she walked by herself
holding God's hand only."

* * *

"Heather was the first person to really make me feel a
part of the family. I can't recall the year but the date
was March 24. Her smile was like sunshine. We were
feeding a church that was visiting Paradise. She said to
me "you need to drink more water". I fell in love with
her right there."

* * *

"She was a joy, was always happy, and never
complained. She loved to talk about her college years -
an uplift to everyone who knew her. She assisted me
during summer camp when I was working with the
finances. Another angel for heavens gain, she will be
missed. God Bless and Prayers."

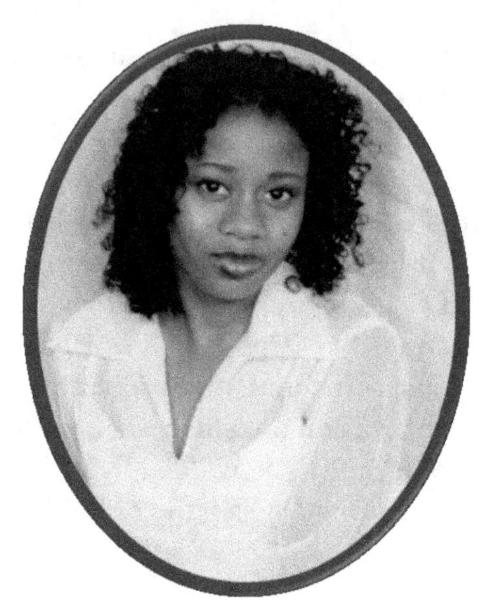

Precious Lord take my hand
Lead me on let me stand
I am tired, I am weak, I am worn
through the storm
through the night
lead me on to the light
precious Lord take my hand
lead me home.

SICKLE CELL ANEMIA

Although Sickle Cell was first described in medical literature almost a century ago there is no known cure. Varying resources quote ranges of 375-600 babies born of African ancestry as carrying the disease. Beyond the Americas' babies born in the Mediterranean, Middle East and India are also affected. In addition, about eight percent of black Americans who do not suffer from the disease itself carry the gene that can be transmitted to their children.

Although more is known about sickle cell disease than about any other inherited disease, no cure for it exists. Sickle cell disease is of enormous social, biological, and historic importance. Improvements during the past two decades in our understanding of the disease and in medical care are permitting those afflicted to live longer, more comfortable and more productive lives.

Ongoing researchers on gene therapy are focusing on whether it may be possible to 'turn off' the action of the gene hemoglobin S that causes sickle cell anemia. Although there is no cure consistent treatment and maintaining overall health can keep many people with Sickle Cell Anemia in reasonably good health. In the past 30 years, life expectancy for sickle cell anemia patients has improved and many now live beyond their 40s and 50s.

The Disease

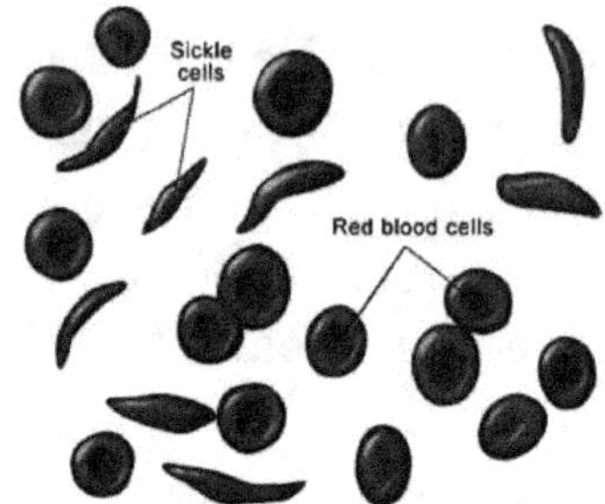

We are not doctors, neither are we specialist, we don't know all the answers, nor do we have all the questions. We can't tell you which battles to choose or which crusades will be won. We can however share a few simple facts we have learned as parents of two children affected by Sickle Cell Anemia disease. Over the years we've amassed a library of amazing resources, a list of highly respected medical professionals, a catalogue of organizations, a few practical tips and a first hand account into the world of this incurable disease.

The internet, your local book store, your medical professional and The Sickle Cell Foundation all have a wealth of information describing this disease. In laymen's terms, Sickle Cell Anemia is a condition in which the body produces red blood cells that are shaped like sickles. Normal red blood cells are disc shaped making it easy for them to flow through the body. Sickle shaped red blood cells cannot move through the body easily, these cells clump and reduce blood flow to the limbs and organs. These cells have a shorter life span than healthy red blood cells.

Sickle Cell is an inherited form of anemia. It is handed down from generation to generation. Normal red blood cells contain the vital protein hemoglobin, which is rich in iron and needed to carry oxygen from the lungs to the entire body. In sickle cell anemia, a mutated gene causes hemoglobin to be defective and causes abnormal development in red blood cells. If you only have one sickle cell gene, it's called sickle cell trait. As we married and prepared to start a family, we learned that we both had one sickle cell gene - (people with the disease are born with two sickle cell genes, one from each parent).

Family planning can be challenging enough – learning that the medical community gives you a 75 to 1 or 25% chance of having a child with Sickle Cell Anemia disease takes family planning to a whole new level. As a family we turned to God. Only he could guide us in making this decision and see us through any trials and tribulations. After a lot of prayers, consultations with professionals, and conversations with family and loved ones, we made an informed decision. Feeling the presence of God and the love of his son Jesus guiding us on this journey, we happily gave birth to our first born, a girl – Heather Anese Burns.

A blood test checking for hemoglobin S (the defective form of hemoglobin underlying Sickle Cell Anemia) confirmed Heather's Sickle Cell Disease. In the United States this blood test is now part of routine newborn screening. Work with your medical professional to determine if your older child or an adult should be tested. The most common symptom of Sickle Cell is the chronic and acute pain attacks. These occur when low oxygen in the body causes the red blood cells to become

rigid and misshapen depriving tissues throughout the
body of much needed oxygen. This can lead to organ
damage, weakened muscles, fatigue, infections, and
strokes. Other symptoms can include:

- Blocked blood vessels or clumps of red blood cells
  in the vessels
- Decrease in the number of red blood cells
- Pain in the organs and joints
- Pain and swelling in the hands and feet
- Damage to the spleen
- Frequent bacterial infections
- Chest pain
- Lung infections such as pneumonia
- Skin ulcers on the lower legs
- Damage to the retina causing vision problems
- Delayed growth and development
- Yellowing of the skin and eyes due to fast
  breakdown of red blood cells
- Confusion or difficulty understanding and
  slurred, garbled or incoherent speech

Known complications of Sickle Cell Anemia Disease

- Stroke - A stroke can occur if the deformed Sickle
  Cells block blood flow to an area of the brain.
  Stroke is one of the most serious complications of
  Sickle Cell Anemia. Signs of a stroke include but
  are not limited to seizures, weakness or
  numbness of arms and legs, sudden speech
  difficulties, and/or loss of consciousness. A stroke
  can be fatal. Seek medical treatment

immediately. Using a specific type of ultrasound (Transcranial), doctors can determine which Sickle Cell Anemia disease carriers have a high risk of stroke

- Acute Chest Syndrome – This life-threatening complication causes chest pain, fever and difficulty breathing. Acute chest syndrome can be caused by a lung infection or Sickle Cell blocking blood vessels in the lungs. Our emergency medical professionals treat with antibiotics, blood transfusions and drugs that opened airways in the lungs - recurrent attacks do damage the lungs. Breathing supplemental oxygen through a breathing mask adds oxygen to the blood and assists in breathing. We have found this to be helpful in cases of Acute Chest Syndrome and/or Sickle Cell crisis.

- Pulmonary Hypertension – About one third of people with Sickle Cell Anemia develop high blood pressure in their lungs (pulmonary hypertension). Shortness of breath and difficulty breathing are common symptoms of this condition. We have been told that Pulmonary Hypertension can ultimately lead to heart failure.

- Organ Damage – Sickle Cells can block blood flow through blood vessels immediately depriving an organ of blood and oxygen. In Sickle Cell Anemia blood can be chronically low on oxygen.

Chronic deprivation of oxygen-rich blood can damage nerves and organs in the body – including but not limited to the kidneys, liver and spleen. Organ damage can be fatal.

- Blindness – Tiny vessels supplying blood to the eyes can get blocked by sickle cells. Over time this can damage the retina – the portion of the eye that processes visual images. This can lead to blindness.

- Gallstones – The breakdown of red blood cells produces a substance called bilirubin. Bilirubin is responsible for yellowing of the skin and eyes (jaundice) in victims of Sickle Cell Anemia. A high level of bilirubin in the body can also lead to gallstones.

BLOOD TRANSFUSIONS

Discussion on the benefits verses the risks of blood transfusions is never ending. Having an informed conversation with your medical provider is crucial. For Sickle Cell Anemia sufferers blood transfusions increase the number of normal red blood cells in circulation – assisting in relieving the anemia. In Sickle Cell Anemia children at a high risk of stroke, regular blood transfusions can decrease that risk. Because blood contains iron, regular blood transfusions can lead to an excessive iron build up. This build up can damage the heart, liver and other essential organs. Deferasirox (Exjade) is an oral medication often used to reduce excess iron levels in patients undergoing regular transfusions.

LIFESTYLE AND IN-HOME REMEDIES

We were blessed with two children, a daughter Heather and a son Keenan. Both were born with the disease Sickle Cell Anemia. On January 24, 2009 Heather died due to complications of Sickle Cell Anemia. Having been blessed with these two wonderful children we knew changing lifestyles, and in-home remedies would be crucial. Things like regular timely childhood vaccinations, yearly flu shots, and immunization against pneumonia to name a few. Over the years there have been a number of lessons learned. Although this list could apply to anyone trying to live a healthy lifestyle, it is crucial for someone challenged with Sickle Cell Anemia disease.

- Take folic acid supplements daily and eat a balanced diet
- Drink plenty of water
- Avoid temperature extremes
- Reduce stress
- Exercise regularly but don't overdo it – listen to your body
- Use over-the-counter medications with caution
- Fly on airplanes with pressurized cabins
- Avoid high-altitude areas

ADULTS

Having both a daughter and son reach adulthood, we feel it is necessary to discuss the struggle with what was formerly known as "Child's Blood Disorder". We have listed referred to sources below however we have incorporated our personal views and opinions in this much needed discussion.

In many ways the problems faced by Sickle Cell patients are simply a reflection of our U.S. Heath Care System which is inadequate in meeting the needs of adults; especially those who have a chronic disease or suffer at the hands of poverty.

Forty years ago the majority of Sickle Cell patients did during childhood - thus primary treatment and care of Sickle Cell patients was focused on the pediatric population. Today there are far more established Sickle Cell specialists in the specialty of pediatrics than there are in the adult realm. In large part this is because only recently has Sickle Cell diseased patients and Sickle Cell Anemia families found themselves living long enough to grow into adulthood.

Both physicians and medical organizations need to increase awareness and create consistent ongoing treatment guidelines for Sickle Cell Anemia and related diseases in the adult population.

Re-hospitalization for adults is high because care for adults isn't as well established as it is for children. One major problem is health care insurance for young adults as they transition out of childhood into adulthood. For many patients, hitting adulthood means loosing guaranteed health care insurance and primary care pediatricians. These young adults are left in transition.

This transition is one of primary concern to the Sickle Cell adult population. Another concern for the adult population is coordination of care. Adult care tends to lack the coordination of care you see in the pediatric community. As parents of two Sickle Cell Anemia diseased adults we have personally experienced the challenges of accessing coordinated medical care.

In closing, if you have a child with sickle cell anemia learn as much as you can about the disease and make sure your child gets the best health care possible. A child with Sickle Cell disease has special needs and requires regular ongoing medical care. As of the day this book went to press, there are no Sickle Cell Centers, or adult doctors trained in the treatment of Sickle Cell Anemia in our home state of Oklahoma. Hopefully by the time you read this, things will have changed.

It is our hope and prayer that by sharing this information and telling our daughter's story, there will be more awareness of the need for improved medical care, better treatment and someday a cure for adults with Sickle Cell Anemia disease

Complications of Sickle Cell Anemia disease both
Heather and Keenan experienced.

Removal of Gall Bladder
Heather age 12
Keenan age 28

Physical Therapy
Heather 2000 - 2005

Strokes
Keenan age 5, 1987
Heather age 24, 2000

Blood Transfusions
Heather and Keenan
Every 4 to 5 weeks

Joint Pain, Swelling Joints
Heather and Keenan

Sickle Cell crisis, Pneumonia, Fever
Heather and Keenan

*Let us run with perseverance the race
marked out for us.*

Hebrews 12:1

EXCHANGE BLOOD TRANSFUSIONS

On January 24, 2009, our daughter Heather died of Acute Chest Syndrome. Had she been treated with "exchange blood transfusions" her life might have been saved. At the time of Heather's death emergency room doctors in our home state failed to offer exchange blood transfusion as a method of treatment for Acute Chest Syndrome in Sickle Cell Patients, although exchange blood transfusions had been around since the mid 1900's and numerous studies had been done on Sickle Cell Diseased patients experiencing Acute Chest Syndrome. The Journal of Pediatrics reported findings from a comparative study as far back as 1995 concluding:

> "Blood transfusion, even simple transfusion of packed erythrocytes, significantly improves oxygenation in children with <u>acute chest syndrome</u> and is a valuable adjunct to therapy"

Children's Medical Center of Brooklyn, State University of New York Health Science Center, USA <u>The Journal of Pediatrics</u> [1995, Comparative Study DOI: 10.1016/S0022-3476(95)70025-0

Paul Swerdlow, MD, Wayne State University reported in the *January 2006 issue of Hematology:*

> "Red cell exchange transfusions remain an effective <u>but possibly underutilized therapy in the acute and chronic treatment of sickle cell disease.</u> In sickle cell disease, increased blood viscosity can cause complications when the hemoglobin exceeds 10 g/dL even if this is due to simple transfusion. Red cell exchange can provide needed oxygen carrying capacity while reducing the overall

viscosity of blood. Acute red cell exchange is useful in acute infarctive stroke, in acute chest and the multi-organ failure syndromes, the right upper quadrant syndrome, and possibly priapism. Neither simple or exchange transfusions are likely to hasten resolution of an acute pain episode."

WikiPedia defines exchange blood transfusion:"
An exchange transfusion is a medical treatment in which apheresis is used to remove one person's red blood cells or platelets and replace them with transfused blood products. Exchange transfusion is used in the treatment of a number of diseases, including: Sickle cell disease. An exchange transfusion requires that the patient's blood be removed and replaced. In most cases, this involves placing one or more thin tubes, called catheters, into a blood vessel. The exchange transfusion is done in cycles: each one usually lasts a few minutes. The patient's blood is slowly withdrawn (usually about 5 to 20 mL at a time, depending on the patient's size and the severity of illness). An equal amount of fresh, prewarmed blood or plasma flows into the patient's body. This cycle is repeated until the correct volume of blood has been replaced. After the exchange transfusion, catheters may be left in place in case the procedure needs to be repeated. In diseases such as sickle cell anemia, blood is removed and replaced with donor blood."

Years before our daughter's death this procedure was saving lives. There are no words to express our frustration and disappointment in learning this "scientifically tested", "internationally practiced" "well known", procedure was available and approved for the treatment of Acute Chest Syndrome in Sickle Cell Patients. Article after article was found on-line and in medical journals referencing studies, results, findings and conclusions. Even the article below directly addresses the benefits of this procedure for Acute Chest Syndrome in Sickle Cell Diseased patients:

"Management of sudden severe illness

Acute chest syndrome, stroke, sepsis, and acute multi-organ failure are leading causes of death in sickle cell disease. A falling hemoglobin value often accompanies these events. Transfusions to improve tissue oxygenation and perfusion are indicated in these seriously ill patients. Controlled clinical trials have not evaluated transfusions in all life-threatening events, but they have become standard medical practice for the events described below:

<u>Acute chest syndrome</u>

When acute chest syndrome is associated with hypoxia and a falling hemoglobin, transfusions are indicated. Studies suggest that early transfusion may prevent the progression of acute pulmonary disease. Since the hemoglobin is low, many patients can be treated with a simple red cell transfusion. In severe cases, exchange blood transfusion / red cell pheresis is recommended."

Recently we have found younger, more recent medical school graduates to be more knowledgeable and better skilled in the treatment of Sickle Cell Diseased adults. Thankfully our son Keenan is receiving this life saving treatment.

Throughout this journey there have been lessons learned. The most important being - get the facts. The better informed you are the better your treatment will be.

In closing, things are changing yet our work as parents, caretakers and medical professionals continues. There are hospitals, clinics and organizations nationwide who are effectively serving Sickle Cell Diseased children and adults. Duke Comprehensive Sickle Cell Center is just one.

"CLINICAL SERVICES

The Duke University Comprehensive Sickle Cell Center is committed to providing the best possible care to patients with sickle cell disease and to finding ways to improve that care. Both in-patient and out-patient care is provided. Medical, surgical, rehabilitative, psychosocial and educational services are provided. The service capacity of the sickle cell center is enhanced through referrals to the vast resources of Duke University Medical Center and the community. Duke University Medical Center has on its staff a number of specialists, such as obstetricians, neurologists, and orthopedic surgeons, who are skilled in working with patients with sickle cell disease. In addition, we offer advanced services for safe blood transfusion and exchange transfusion of patients with sickle cell disease when such services are required."

SICKLE CELL ORGANIZATIONS

There are numerous entities doing research, providing medical care, supporting families and raising awareness about Sickle Cell Disease. These entities usually call themselves organizations, "associations", "foundations" or "groups".   Most are state based and non-profit - providing services to patients within a specific mile radius. One of the largest nationwide organizations is the Sickle Cell Disease Association of America (SCDAA) formed in 1971.

"The vision for a national coordinated approach to addressing issues related to sickle cell disease was unveiled in 1971 when representatives of 15 community sickle cell organizations met at "Wingspread," a Racine, Wisconsin conference center, as guest of the Johnson Foundation. Out of that meeting, the National Association for Sickle Cell Disease was created. The name was changed to Sickle Cell Disease Association of America, Inc. in. 1994."

scdaa@sicklecelldisease.org,
www.sicklecelldisease.org

Many of these groups or organizations fall under the realm of a 501(c) non-profit organization or are a United Way organization. Although their names may vary most have the same goals – raising awareness of and supporting the Sickle Cell Anemia patient and their families.

With the advent of the internet finding the support you need has been made easy. There are hundreds of websites providing current information on physicians, hospitals, and support groups in your area. Many of these groups also offer child care, day camps, recreation facilities, educational programs and screening.

Unfortunately many communities don't get the support they need to fund these programs. Others fail to offer any assistance at all. It is up to you, the citizens of your communities, cities and states to make your voices heard. Sickle Cell Anemia is primarily common in people whose families or ancestors come from Saudi Arabia, India, Caribbean islands, South or Central America, or Africa. However more recently people of Mediterranean ancestry; Turkey, Italy, and Greece, have been found to carry the gene.

As you can see we have not suggested any specific doctor, hospital, organization, or facility. Facing the challenges of discovering you carry the Sickle Cell gene, or learning that someone you love has the disease can be devastating. We are simply sharing some of the information we've gathered living as a Sickle Cell Anemia family for over 30 years. Your medical professional is your primary source of knowledge. In some states your United Way or Public Health Department can also provide assistance. The more knowledge you have about Sickle Cell, the happier your life and the life of your loved ones will be.

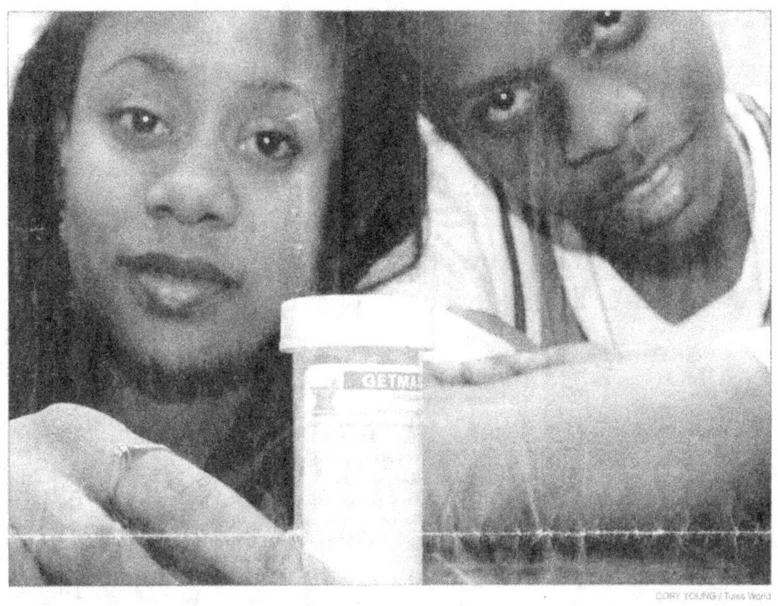

CORY YOUNG / Tulsa World

Siblings Heather (left) and Keenan Burns live with sickle-cell disease. They look to each other for strength as they fight the disease.

Thicker than water

Brother, sister refuse to give up as they fight sickle-cell anemia together

*"I am not going to lie, some days are
really hard, but there are some
that are so good you forget
you are sick"*

71

OUR HEROES HEATHER AND KEENAN

"There will always be people who suffer
with more severe illnesses and more
grueling challenges. Consider the extent
of your blessings and say a daily
prayer for these people."

Doctors say it is rare for both siblings to have Sickle
Cell Anemia disease when both parents carry the gene.
Normally only one in four offspring within the same
family is affected. Heather and Keenan are the medical
rarity that makes our family special. Their passion for
life, heartfelt laughter, and enjoyment for all things
comical makes coping with this illness easier to handle.

"Heather, Keenan and an all-powerful God
The wind beneath our wings"

Our heroes Heather and Keenan moved into their own
apartments in 2005; gaining their own independence –
living as adults with this fatal disease. Taking
advantage of life and all it had to offer. Placing
themselves and their futures, in the hands of an
almighty God.

"Courage doesn't always roar,
sometimes courage is the
quiet voice at the end
of the day saying,
I will try again tomorrow."

"One of our goals, every step of the way is to prepare our
children for independence – to leave the nest. We
believe there is a balance in life for everyone no matter
what odds have befallen on you - you can do what
anyone else does"
- Patricia A. Burns

"We're trying to make their lives
the best they can be"
- Sam A. Burns

"When Keenan and I were both in the hospital
and had beds side by side, I was so upset and kept
saying, why me? Why me? But Keenan didn't do
that, and he had it worse than I do."
- Heather A. Burns

"When she went to the hospital I told her that it was
going to be all right and that she was going to make it
through. God is with you and don't give up"
- Keenan A. Burns

RESOURCES

Rettner, Rachel, "What is Sickle Cell Disease?"
Live Science, 2011, Article 30 July 2010,
www.livescience.com/6805-sickle-cell-disease.html

"Adults Struggle With What Used To Be Child's
Blood Disorder" Live Science 2011, 1 Aug. 2010
http://www.livescience.com/6815-adults-struggle-
child-blood-disorder.html

By Mayo Clinic Staff "Definition – Sickle Cell
Anemia", © 1998-2012, Mayo Foundation for Medical
Education and   Research,
www.mayoclinic.com/health/sickle-cell-
anemia/DS00324

"Sickle Cell Anemia", Diseases and Conditions
Cleveland Clinic, The Cleveland Clinic © 1995-2011
http://my.clevelandclinic.org/disorders/Sickle_Cell_A
nemia/hic_Sickle_Cell_Anemia.aspx

Dr. Noreen A. Kassam, "Dr. Noreen A. Kassam Disscusses
the Inherited Disease Which is More Likely to Effect Ethnic
Minorities", Issue 70, July 2010, © emel media limited
Registered England and Wales. No. 4745601,
http://www.emel.com/article?id=74&a_id=2060

There are many more in-print, and on-line resources
of Sickle Cell Anemia symptoms, causes, risk factors,
complications, treatments and tests. You can also find
complication preventions and ways to stay healthy.

By JASON ASHLEY WRIGHT World Scene Writer,
Published: 10/10/2011

INAUGURAL EVENT TO BENEFIT
MEMORIAL SCHOLARSHIP

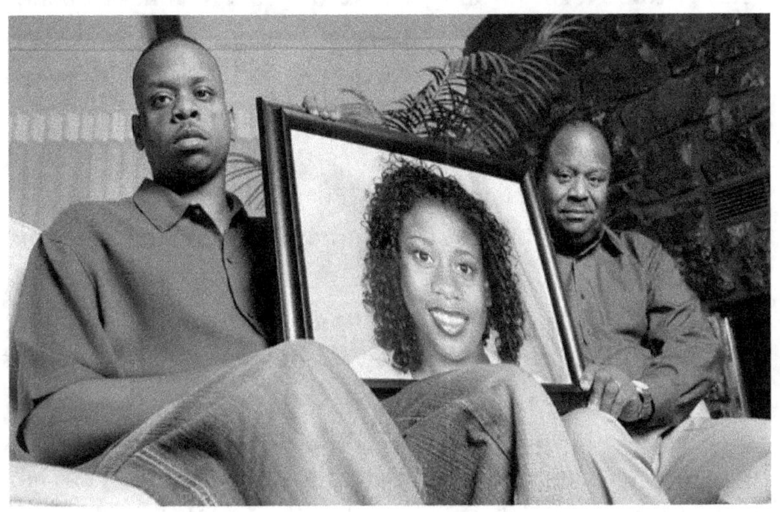

Sam Burns (right) and his son, Keenan Burns, hold
a photo at their home in Tulsa of Heather Burns,
who died of sickle cell disease. The Burns family
has started a foundation that will award
scholarships to students who have life-altering
diseases or face financial hardships.

MICHAEL WYKE / Tulsa World Article

By JASON ASHLEY WRIGHT, Published: 10/10/2011

"Heaven and Earth shall pass away but my words
shall not pass away.", Mark 13:31.

That Bible verse was printed on cards that Heather
Burns would hand out as part of her personal ministry.
"She just believed in the word and that the Lord's word
could see her through anything," said her father, Sam
Burns. She was intelligent, outgoing, never met a
stranger, said Patricia Burns, her mother.

"She let her light shine since preschool," Patricia
Burns said. Perhaps most evident, Heather had a strong
faith, one that remained unshaken through her struggle
with complications stemming from sickle cell anemia,
which claimed her life January. 24, 2009.

"It seemed to give her fortitude, the courage to aspire
to grow, to keep going," Patricia Burns said. It's her
faith that inspired her family to forge the Heather
Burns Memorial Scholarship Fund, a nonprofit
organization the Burns family formed earlier this year.
The group will host its inaugural 5K walk at 9:30 a.m.
Oct. 22 starting at 900 N. Greenwood Ave.

As active as she was, Heather would've liked the 5K
fundraiser, her family said. "She would always run
home, saying, 'I want to do this, I want to do that,"
Patricia Burns said, "She just had a zeal. It was a
passion she had within her."

When Patricia and Sam were students at Langston University, they had a blood test that revealed they each carried the sickle cell trait, Sam said. If two people have the trait and pass it on, there's a 1 in 4 chance their child will have the disease. "In our minds, we thought our odds would be a little better," Sam said. But about six months after Heather's birth, they discovered she had sickle cell. About five years later, they had their son, Keenan, who also has sickle cell.

The disease affects red blood cells, which carry oxygen through the body, Sam Burns explained. The name of the disease is derived from the cells, which are normally rounded, when some take on the curved-blade shape of a sickle. Consequently, the cells aren't able to deliver as much oxygen throughout the body. Growing up, Heather and Keenan were on daily penicillin, Sam Burns said. They also had to be careful not to become too hot or too cold, as extreme temperatures could make them sick. Heather didn't let it stop her, though. She was a cheerleader at Will Rogers High School then attended University of Oklahoma Langston University and earned a Associate's Degree in Mass Communications from Northeastern Oklahoma A&M College in Miami. Further education was cut short when Heather suffered a debilitating stroke in 2000. Almost paralyzed and barely able to walk, Heather went through rehabilitation therapy at St. John Medical Center.

As she progressed through therapy and strived for greater independence, Heather wanted to drive, Sam Burns said. They arranged for her to visit the University of Central Oklahoma, where she lived on campus for a month while learning to operate a specially outfitted car. Eventually, she moved into her own apartment. "She was getting there," Sam said. "She was definitely making progress toward getting back to school. She really put a lot of value on being able to get her undergraduate degree." But on a Friday in late January, Heather complained of chest pains and had trouble breathing, her father recalled. She was experiencing acute chest syndrome, the leading cause of death among patients with sickle cell disease, according to the New England Journal of Medicine. Heather's family took her to the hospital that evening and, on that Saturday night she died.

To honor their daughter's memory, the Burns family wanted to create a scholarship fund to help students who not only suffer with sickle cell but also face other physical, mental, social and economical challenges that stand in their way of pursuing higher education. The first scholarship will be awarded later this month. "We know she would applaud that," Patricia Burns said when asked how Heather would react to a scholarship in her name. "She put her faith in God, and that carried her through," her mother said. "The scriptures tell us he will never leave us or forsake us, and he will be there for us in our time of need".

For more about the Heather Burns Memorial Scholarship Fund, call 918-582-1515, or visit tulsaworld.com/hbmsf

TULSA WORLD
By JASON ASHLEY WRIGHT World Scene Writer,
Published: 10/10/2011

Into adulthood, sickle cell patients rely on ER

by Julia Evangelou Strait , December 10, 2012

Patients with sickle cell disease rely more on the emergency room as they move from pediatric to adult health care, according to researchers at Washington University School of Medicine in St. Louis. An analysis of Medicaid data of more than 3,200 patients with sickle cell disease shows that emergency room visits tripled from age 15 to age 24. The research is reported Dec. 10 at the American Society of Hematology's annual meeting in Atlanta. "There seems to be a breakdown in medical care during the transition from childhood to adulthood," says hematologist Morey A. Blinder, MD, associate professor of medicine. "Not only emergency department usage, but hospitalizations go up during this time as well."

One possible explanation for the increased reliance on emergency care, according to Blinder, is the relative lack of adult health care providers with experience caring for sickle cell patients. Similar issues are arising for other pediatric diseases, such as cystic fibrosis and hemophilia, which were previously fatal. Over the past few decades, an increasing number of children and teenagers are living into adulthood with these conditions and there often aren't enough primary care physicians who can provide care for these adult patients. Sickle cell disease refers to a number of inherited genetic conditions that cause the normally round, disk-like red blood cells to take on a characteristic "sickle" shape. These malformed red blood cells do not carry oxygen to the body as well as healthy cells and are prone to clogging smaller blood vessels. The condition is often painful in places the cells block blood flow.

Some of the more severe complications include blindness, strokes and pneumonia. In the study, researchers examined data of 3,200 Medicaid patients with sickle cell disease from the mid 1990s through 2010. The researchers followed patients from five states (Florida, New Jersey, Missouri, Iowa and Kansas) for an average of six years each and included those moving from pediatric to adult care. The study showed that emergency department visits tripled over nine years, increasing from 0.76 per quarter at age 15 to more than two per quarter at age 24. At age 36, use of emergency care peaked at almost three visits per quarter, or about one per month. Even by age 50, reliance on emergency care did not return to the lower levels seen in childhood. More emergency care and hospitalizations also result in higher overall medical costs. Total health care costs were more than $7,000 higher per quarter for patients making heavier use of the emergency department, even as they tended to spend less on medication, perhaps simply failing to fill prescriptions.

Blinder says the St. Louis region and Missouri in general have good support for adults with sickle cell disease, though this is not always the case nationally. "In areas without good adult support for this disease, you have to identify adult physicians who would be interested in treating sickle cell patients," Blinder says. "They could be hematologists or even internists, but in general there are not enough providers for adult sickle cell patients. This study highlights an emerging problem in transitioning pediatric age patients to adulthood, and the need to explore new ways to facilitate that process," Blinder says. The study was funded by Novartis Pharmaceuticals. Blinder is a consultant for Novartis and receives some research support from the company. Several of the study's co-investigators are employed by Novartis.

Blinder MA, Vekeman F, Sasane M, Trahey A, Paley C, Magestro M, Duh MS. Age-related emergency department reliance and healthcare resource utilization in patients with sickle cell disease. Presented Dec. 10, 2012, American Society of Hematology Annual Meeting.

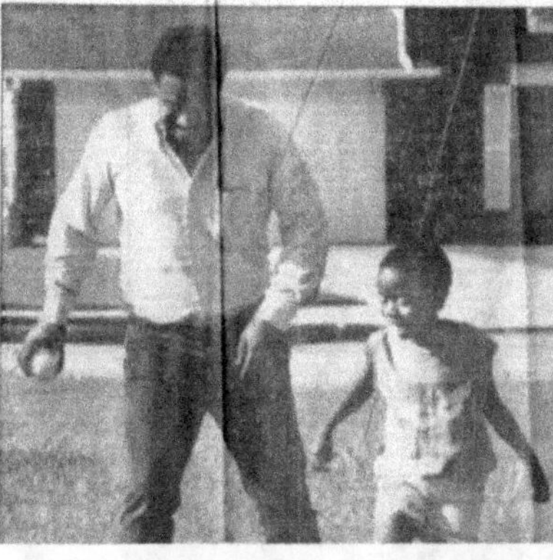

Family winning battle with disease

Until the year 2000, The Tulsa Tribune is following the lives of 21 children who began school in 1997 in the same kindergarten class at Barnard Elementary School.

Today, the focus is on one pupil who has a serious disease.

Stories by MELINDA MORRIS
The Tulsa Tribune

In preschool, Keenan Burns could write his name with ease.

But about midway through kindergarten, Keenan was struggling to form the 11 letters that make up his name while his classmates were learning to put together sentences.

"It was frustrating for him," said his father, Sam Burns. "I don't know if he knew why he couldn't do it anymore."

Keenan still knew what the letters were, but a minor stroke, brought on by sickle cell anemia, had hurt his ability to do things such as write as legibly as he once did.

Now, 1½ years after the stroke, Keenan's parents say he loves to write, put together puzzles and play on his father's computer. The improvements, they say, are because of prayer, good nutrition and care, and moving him from a crowded class to a smaller one.

Sickle cell anemia is an inherited disease. Neither Burns nor his wife, Patricia, are affected, but both carry the sickle cell trait and knew they had a 1 in 4 chance of having a child with the disease.

The disease causes the normally doughnut-shaped red blood cells to become sickle shaped.

"Instead of little round 'doughnuts' that pass through (the blood system) smoothly, the sickle cells jam up," Burns said.

The blockages cause sickle cell anemia "crises," pain attacks that can strike any part of the body and may require hospitalization.

Keenan began showing symptoms of sickle

Awarness sought for sickle cell

Yes, sickle cell anemia mostly strikes black people.

But advocates for awareness of the genetic blood disorder say blacks are not the only ones who should care, and much more research and many more services are needed.

Sickle cell anemia causes the normally round blood cells to become sickle-shaped, which can cause anemia and sickle cell "crises."

A sickle cell crisis, or pain attack, occurs when sickle-shaped cells bunch up in blood vessels and prevent oxygen from reaching tissues and organs. The disease can shorten lives by half, although experts say there is no set life expectancy.

"Some people think it's only a disease of black people, but it's also a disease of Mediterranean people," said Sam Burns, former board president of the Oklahoma chapter of the National Association for Sickle Cell Disease Foundation.

People of Spanish, Greek, Italian, Turkish, Asian and Indian descent also may have the dis

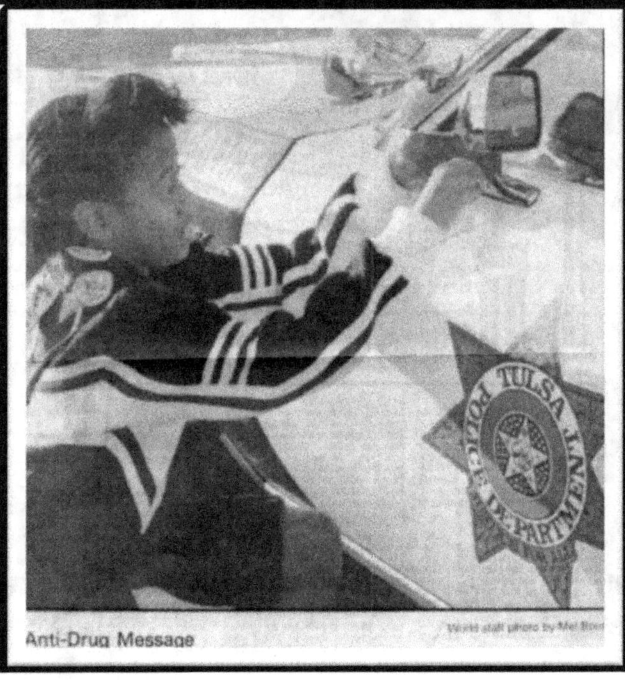

Anti-Drug Message

World staff photo by Mel Bor

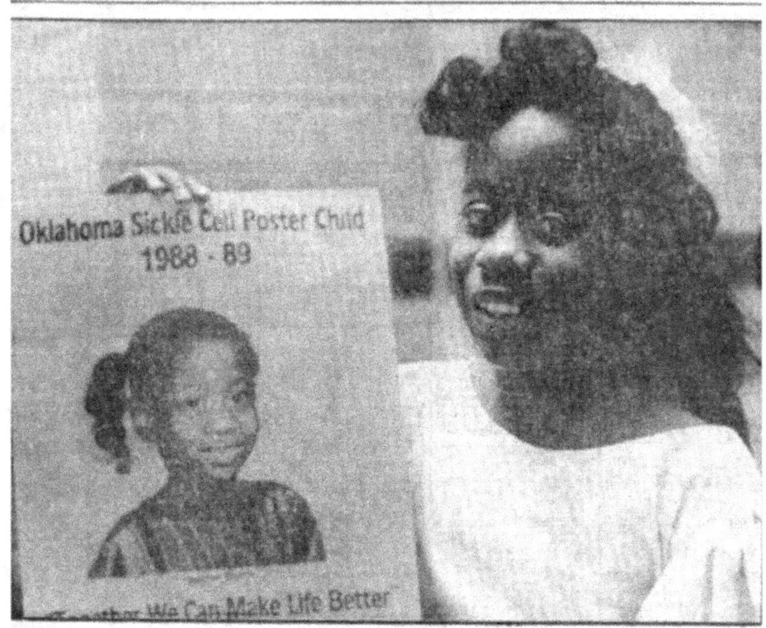

World Staff Photo by Steve Crane

Model Child

Heather Burns, 11, is the 1988 Oklahoma Sickle Cell Anemia Poster Child. The Carver Middle School sixth-grader was introduced Friday. September has been named Sickle Cell Anemia Awareness month in the state.

September is Sickle Cell month

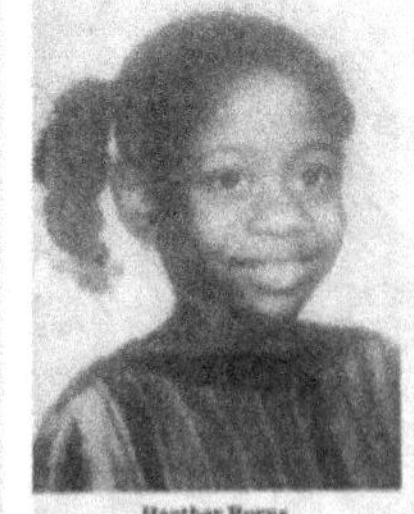

Heather Burns

The Oklahoma Sickle Cell Anemia Research Foundation, Inc. (OSCARFI) has set its activities for National Sickle Cell Month. The Calendar of Events are as follows:

An Educational Seminar to be held September 16th at the Sheraton Century in Oklahoma City; a Casino Night Fund-raiser the night of September 16th in Oklahoma City,

and an Openhouse including an Art Show and sale to be held September 25th at Westview Med Clinic 3606 N. Cinncinati in Tulsa. The annual fund-raiser in Tulsa will be a Mediterranean Evening Dinner Dance, September 30, at University Center at Tulsa, 700 North Greenwood. The evening will feature Mediterreanean food live entertainment; dress for the occasion is optional. Tickets are available by contacting OSCARFI.

Heather Burns a 6th grade student at Carver Middle School is the 1988 poster child of the year for the State of Oklahoma. She is the daughter of Sam and Patricia Burns of Tulsa, and the granddaughter of Thelma Burns, a retired school teacher.

OSCARFI was founded in 1971 and has been serving the Tulsa community through education screening, and counseling. organization has screen (statistics). The state organization is now operating Oklahoma City and is expanding efforts throughout the State.

For information about Sickle Anemia or to schedule screening the disease, contact OSCARF 428-1974. Executive Director OSCARFI is Mable Rice. Sh Johnston, R. N., M. S., Preside the Board of Directors.

HEATHER'S FAVORITES

Joshua 1:5

⁵There shall not any man be able to stand before thee all
the days of thy life: as I was with Moses, so I will be
with thee: I will not fail thee, nor forsake thee.

Galatians 4:9

⁹But now, after that ye have known God, or rather
are known of God, how turn ye again to the weak
and beggarly elements, whereunto ye desire again
to be in bondage?

Matthew 17:1-8

¹And after six days Jesus taketh Peter, James, and John
his brother, and bringeth them up into an high
mountain apart, ²And was transfigured before them:
and his face did shine as the sun, and his raiment was
white as the light. ³And, behold, there appeared unto
them Moses and Elias talking with him. ⁴Then
answered Peter, and said unto Jesus, Lord, it is good for
us to be here: if thou wilt, let us make here three
tabernacles; one for thee, and one for Moses, and one for
Elias. ⁵While he yet spake, behold, a bright cloud
overshadowed them: and behold a voice out of the cloud,
which said, This is my beloved Son, in whom I am well
pleased; hear ye him. ⁶And when the disciples heard it,
they fell on their face, and were sore afraid. ⁷And Jesus
came and touched them, and said, Arise, and be not
afraid. ⁸And when they had lifted up their eyes, they
saw no man, save Jesus only.

Mark 13:31

³¹Heaven and earth shall pass away:
but my words shall not pass away.

Ephesians 4:22-24

22 that you put off, concerning your former conduct, the old man which grows corrupt according to the deceitful lusts, 23 and be renewed in the spirit of your mind, 24 and that you put on the new man which was created according to God, in true righteousness and holiness.

Galatians 5:22-23

22But the fruit of the Spirit is love, joy, peace, longsuffering, gentleness, goodness, faith, 23Meekness, temperance: against such there is no law.

Philippians 4:8

8Finally, brethren, whatsoever things are true, whatsoever things are honest, whatsoever things are just, whatsoever things are pure, whatsoever things are lovely, whatsoever things are of good report; if there be any virtue, and if there be any praise, think on these things.

John 14:1-3

1Let not your heart be troubled: ye believe in God, believe also in me. 2In my Father's house are many mansions: if it were not so, I would have told you. I go to prepare a place for you. 3And if I go and prepare a place for you, I will come again, and receive you unto myself; that where I am, there ye may be also.

Philippians 4:13

13I can do all things through Christ which strengthened me.

Psalm 100

[1]Make a joyful noise unto the LORD, all ye lands. [2]Serve
the LORD with gladness: come before his presence with
singing. [3]Know ye that the LORD he is God: it is he
that hath made us, and not we ourselves; we are his
people, and the sheep of his pasture. [4]Enter into his
gates with thanksgiving, and into his courts with praise:
be thankful unto him, and bless his name. [5]For the
LORD is good; his mercy is everlasting; and his truth
endureth to all generations.

II Timothy 3:16

All scripture is given by inspiration of God,
and is profitable for doctrine,
for reproof, for correction,
for instruction in righteousness.

Our Father
Which art in Heaven
Hallowed be thy name.
Thy kingdom come,
Thy will be done in earth,
as it is in heaven.
Give us this day our daily bread.
And forgive us our debts,
as we forgive our debtors.
And lead us not into temptation,
but deliver us from evil:
For thine is the kingdom,
and the power, and the glory,
for ever.
Amen

The Burns Family,
Samuel, Patricia, and Keenan
Thank you for sharing our amazing journey.
We are truly Blessed.

ACKNOWLEDGEMENTS

We give thanks, praise and glory to God. We are grateful and humble for God directing our path, protecting us and granting us grace and mercy. We give thanks to God for blessing us with our children Heather and Keenan. We would like to acknowledge the following people, individuals, groups and organizations who have given support, encouragement, service, love and prayers. Our parents Heather and Keenan's grandparents, Samuel A. Burns Sr., Thelma Thompson Burns, John Wesley House Sr., and Jeannette Hardeman House. All the aunts, uncles, cousins, nieces, nephews, friends, ministers, church members, Rev Leroy Jordan, Sunday School teachers, youth leaders, high school choir director, Girl Scout Sponsors, people in the community, teachers/counselors, Cheer Leader Sponsors, the Sickle Cell Organization of Tulsa, the Sickle Cell Center @Emory University, Dr. William Geffen, nurse Shelly Prather, Dr. Anita Christopher, Dr. Jihad Khattab, nurse Cindy Divers, the Oklahoma Eagle newspaper, graphic designers Linda Murphy and Stephanie Busby, , Mrs. Mabel Rice, all the doctors and nurses, the Heather Burns Memorial Scholarship Fund Board members, Heather's cousin Sharon Harris for the beautiful poems, Mrs. Denise Mason CPA, and Shirley Howard Hall for writing and editing. We would humbly like to acknowledge ourselves for being "obedient to complete praise".

When you are sorrowful,
look again in your heart
And you shall see that in truth
you are weeping for that
which has been your delight.

Gibran

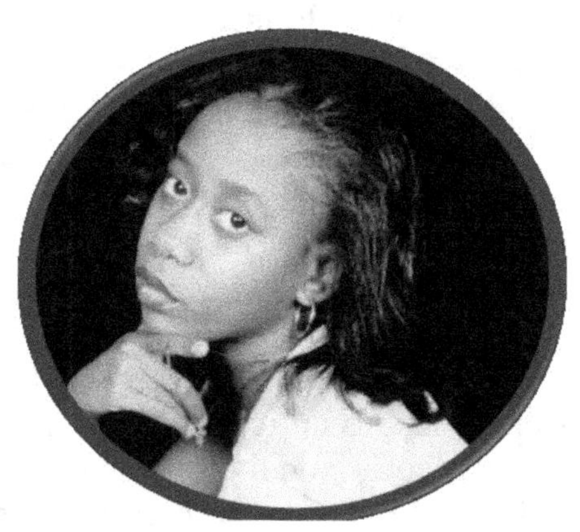

About the Authors

Patricia Burns was born in Langston Oklahoma. A 1972 graduate of Langston University with a Bachelors of Arts in Education, she completed her Masters of Education and Counseling degree, (plus thirty) at Northeastern State University. A teacher and counselor in Tulsa Public Schools, her lifelong career in education ended with her retirement in 2001. Church and community activities include Vice President of Paradise Baptist Church, Sunday school teacher, church choir, Missionary Society, Tulsa Urban League Guild, and worked with Mrs. Mabel Rice *(former executive director of the Sickle Cell Anemia Association)* in the founding of the first Sickle Cell Anemia Support Group in Tulsa, Oklahoma. She continues work in her church, as an advocate in the Sickle Cell Community, and is Chairperson of the Heather Burns Memorial Scholarship Fund. She discovered she carried the Sickle Cell Trait, in 1973.

Samuel A. Burns Jr. was born in Tuskegee, Alabama. He attended secondary and high school in Tulsa Oklahoma and in 1971, graduated from Langston University with a Bachelor of Science degree in Business Administration with a major in Accounting. Church and community activities include Church Treasurer, Trustee, Sunday school teacher, church choir, church brotherhood, Tulsa Urban League, YMCA, and in 1987 and 1988 he served as president of the Tulsa Chapter Sickle Cell Anemia Association.

An active Alpha Phi Alpha he has held the office of, Vice President, Treasurer and Financial Secretary. A career in sales ended in June 2012 when he retired from the Hilti Corporation. Sam continues to work in his church and community and is President of the Heather Burns Memorial Scholarship Fund. He discovered he carried the Sickle Cell Trait in 1973. In 1971 Sam and Patricia married. They currently reside in Tulsa Oklahoma

The Burns family, Samuel, Patricia, Heather and Keenan were named "Outstanding Church Family" while attending First Baptist Church North Tulsa.

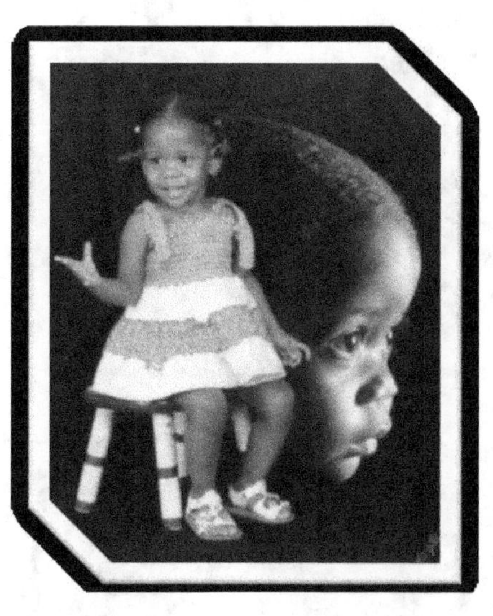

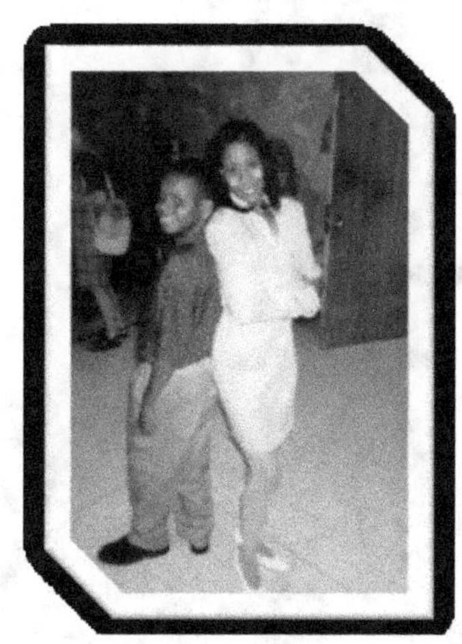

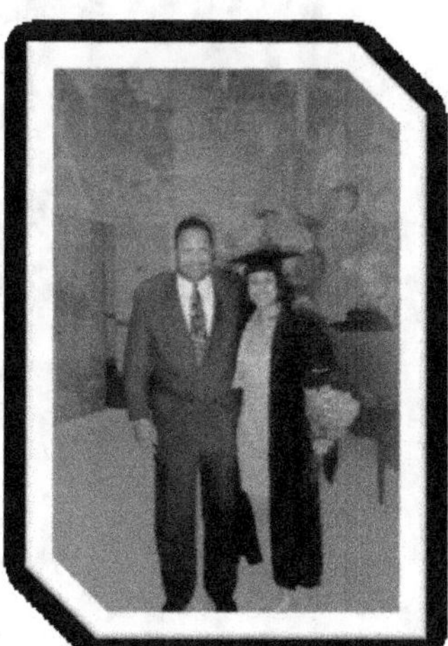

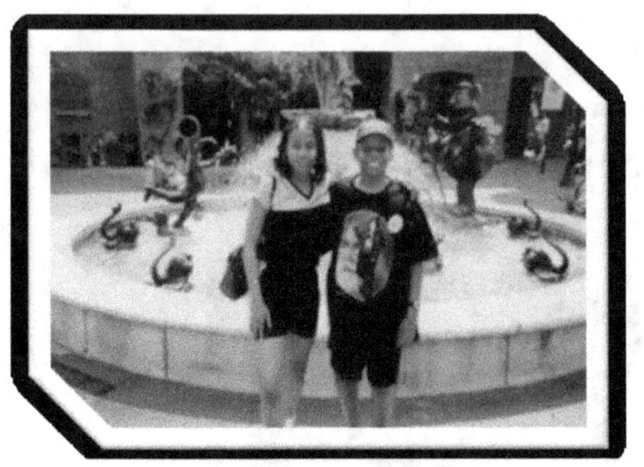

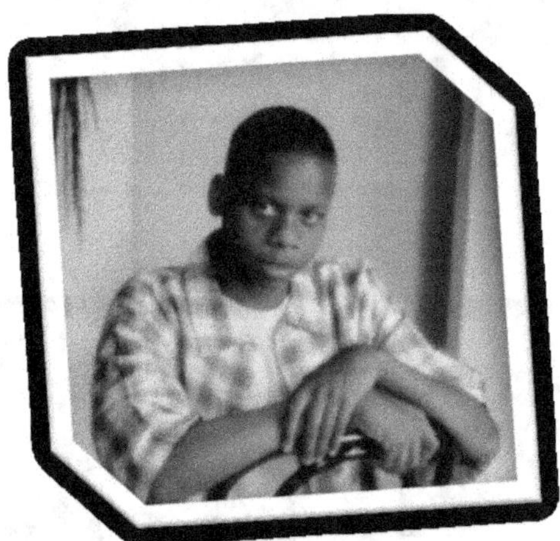

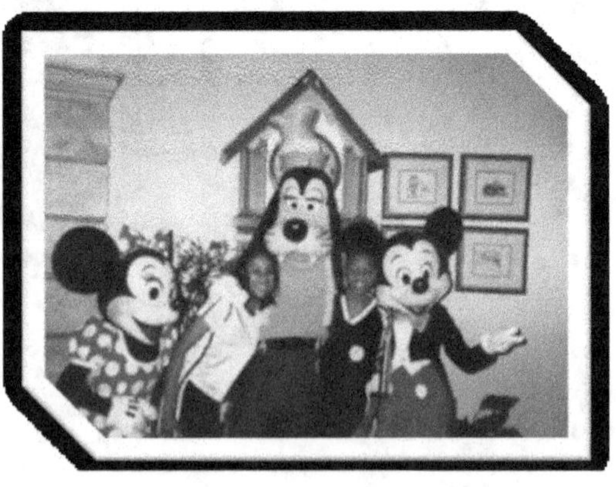

THE HEATHER BURNS
MEMORIAL SCHOLARSHIP FUND

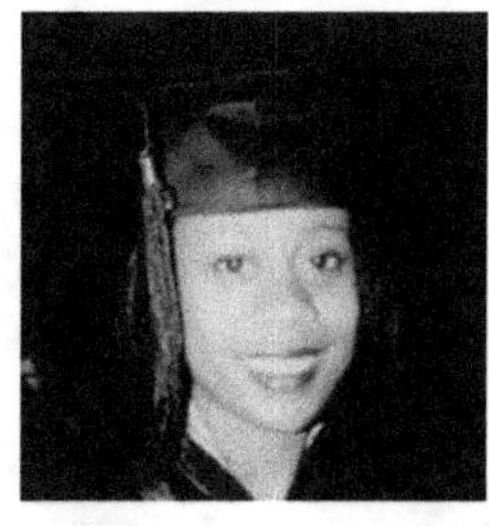

When Heather passed away from complications of Sickle Cell Anemia disease a group of family, relatives and friends came together to form the Heather Burns Memorial Scholarship Fund. To honor Heather's appreciation for higher education, the fund was created to help students with Sickle Cell Anemia Disease, life threatening diseases, and financial hardships attend a college/university, or other school of higher learning.

Heather Burns Memorial Scholarship Fund is a 501(c)(3) nonprofit scholarship program. Donations to the organization provide financial assistance to qualified students. Students can apply for the scholarship by downloading the application from the organization's website at www.hbmsf.org. Students applying for the scholarship must hold or expect to hold acceptance to an accredited college/university or other school of higher learning

Donations to the organization can be made by visiting our website at: www.hbmsf.org/donations.html

For further information contact:
Sam Burns Jr., President
Heather Burns Memorial Scholarship Fund
Email: sburns@hbmsf.org
www.hbmsf.org

www.ingramcontent.com/pod-product-compliance
Lightning Source LLC
Chambersburg PA
CBHW070814240726
48654CB00007B/343